"Megan Febuary's Br̲~~~~~~ tive, self-reflective wo̲~~~ ~~~~~~ ~~ ~~~~ ~~~~~~~ ~~~ ~~~~~~~. This well-researched, beautifully written, and deeply genuine book allows readers to consider the stories locked inside their bodies and empowers them to get the words on the page. February is a loving witness and gentle guide through the various obstacles that keep so many of us from healing, writing, and truly living. Part craft book, part memoir, and part dispatch from the gentle heart of someone who's done her own deep work, *Brave the Page* will be an invaluable resource for anyone interested in the glorious work of healing through writing."

Christie Tate, *New York Times* bestselling author of *GROUP: How One Therapist and a Circle of Strangers Saved My Life* and *B.F.F.: A Memoir of Friendship Lost and Found*

"With a depth of knowledge, an abiding sense of compassion, and the practical tools of a wise teacher, Megan Febuary's *Brave the Page* lovingly guides readers through the process of writing their stories with dignity, grace, and care. This book will be of deep support to all who are looking to explore more human, embodied ways of sharing their stories on the page."

Lisa Olivera, author of *Already Enough*

"Megan Febuary's tour de force of writing compels us to imagine our story as a world worth creating and honoring through the touch of a keyboard or a pen. Writing is a holy, liminal space where more truth can be engaged in reading what we wrote than merely speaking it out loud. Megan's lifegiving prose is poetry for the soul. This powerful book will help you reclaim your life through the power of putting your story into words."

Dan B. Allender, PhD, professor of counseling psychology and founding president, The Seattle School of Theology and Psychology

"Megan reminds us that we are the authors of our own lives. A liberating and compassionate exploration of the radical power of putting words to the page."

Aime McNee, author of *We Need Your Art*

"In *Brave the Page*, Megan Febuary reminds us that our stories—especially the hard ones—are worth telling. Her personal journey, paired with practical tools, invites readers to explore the depths of their own stories and find healing through writing. It's a powerful, soul-stirring guide and a beautiful testament to the healing power of storytelling, one that will resonate deeply with anyone seeking to transform their pain into something meaningful and empowering."

Lisa Weinert, author of *Narrative Healing: Awaken the Power of Your Story*

"Megan Febuary's work with Women Who Roar has always been a force for empowerment, and her new book *Brave the Page* continues that mission with grace and wisdom. It made me feel truly guided and supported on my current creative journey. This is the kind of book I would love to hand out to writers, creative friends, and students as an invaluable guide for their own paths. Megan's vision shines through every page, offering encouragement and insight to all who seek to find their voice."

Sabrina Ward Harrison, author of *Spilling Open: The Art of Becoming Yourself*

BRAVE THE PAGE

BRAVE
THE PAGE

HOW WRITING OUR HARD STORIES
BRINGS HEALING AND WHOLENESS

MEGAN FEBUARY

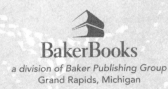

BakerBooks

a division of Baker Publishing Group
Grand Rapids, Michigan

Published by Baker Books
a division of Baker Publishing Group
Grand Rapids, Michigan
BakerBooks.com

Printed in the United States of America

Library of Congress Cataloging-in-Publication Data
Names: Febuary, Megan, author.
Title: Brave the page : how writing our hard stories brings healing and wholeness / Megan Febuary.
Description: Grand Rapids, Michigan : Baker Books, a division of Baker Publishing Group, [2025] | Includes bibliographical references.
Identifiers: LCCN 2024038999 | ISBN 9781540904775 (paperback) | ISBN 9781540904980 (casebound) | ISBN 9781493450459 (ebook)
Subjects: LCSH: Creative writing—Therapeutic use. | Creative writing—Psychological aspects. | Autobiography—Therapeutic use. | Memory. | Healing.
Classification: LCC RC489.W75 F43 2023 | DDC 615.8/5163—dc23/eng/20241021
LC record available at https://lccn.loc.gov/2024038999

Cover design by Derek Thornton, Notch Design

Published in association with The Bindery Agency, www.TheBinderyAgency.com.

Baker Publishing Group publications use paper produced from sustainable forestry practices and postconsumer waste whenever possible.

25 26 27 28 29 30 31   7 6 5 4 3 2 1

To every person who has walked
the long, dark halls
in search of your stories
and the truths they hold.
May your journey inward
lead you closer to the words
that have been hard to find
and to the healing you have longed for.

CONTENTS

As your tears fall over that wounded place,
May they wash away your hurt and free your heart.
May your forgiveness still the hunger of the wound

So that, for the first time, you can walk away from that place,
Reunited with your banished heart, now healed and freed,
And feel the clear, free air bless your new face.

John O'Donohue, "For Someone Awakening
to the Trauma of His or Her Past"

HELLO, BODY

Our bodies are storytellers, holding the pages of our lives inside. Some pages are tucked away in drawers we've forgotten about. Some pages have been crumpled up, burned, and put through the shredder; but still, they are there in our bodies, even if we can't see them. So much of the healing process is about uncovering these displaced pages that have formed us over the years so we can begin transforming those fragmented stories into a cohesive whole.

My body first began speaking to me when I was twelve years old. I was diagnosed with scleroderma, a rare autoimmune disease that creates discolored patches and hardening of the skin caused by an overproduction of collagen in the connective tissue. In general, I was asymptomatic. You would never even know I had this disease—until I put on a swimsuit. The dark discoloration on my arms and legs made it look as though I had bruises all over my body. Sometimes the other kids would cry out, "What happened to you? Somebody beating you up at home?" Those were the last days I wore shorts. I exchanged all my summer clothes for winter ones. While most of my classmates wore cutoff shorts and tank tops, I layered myself in baggy jeans that hung loose on my hips and sweaters that covered nearly every inch of my skin, turning myself into a sweaty puddle in the humid Louisiana heat.

So, in middle school, when life is a season of firsts—first kiss, first dance, first zit, first tampon—I also experienced my first illness. We visited several doctors who were clueless about this rare disease, but at last I was seen by a specialist who had moppy black hair and wore thick-framed glasses. He smelled like musty penicillin—something sour with a hint of mold. With my parents gathered around in a small hospital room, he used a magnifying glass under sharp fluorescent light to investigate my strange skin, taking pictures and notes to share with other doctors about this diagnosis. I felt like a lab rat on display, but a necessary one to study and understand.

Following my diagnosis, my family and friends searched the internet and ugly-cried over the images they found: a series of gaunt faces, shrunken mouths, gnarled bones, and disfigured frames. I looked down at my skin. I could see the outward damage, but I felt completely fine on the inside. It didn't match the frenzy from others I was experiencing, as if the disease was dislocated in me and I in it.

I can't tell you where the feelings about my diagnosis existed in my body around this time, perhaps hidden somewhere with the other emotions I was unsure how to manage. I suppose everyone handles their feelings differently—my mom clung close, my dad's eyes were fixed in worry, my best friend sobbed, my brothers were remote, my grandparents prayed in staunch devotion, and I, well, I took long walks along the levee by our house and in the ditches like I had done when I was smaller and things felt easy.

In the second year after my diagnosis, my family went on a trip to West Virginia to visit my grandparents, who were part of a small Church of God evangelical church that sat high in the Blue Ridge Mountains. I had been to church services before, but never one quite like this. The chapel was small and hot, with crowded pews stretching across both sides. I watched as women filled their familiar seats, beehive hairdos set high on their heads. They bobbled up and down in agreement with confident shouts of "Amen!" and "Hallelujah!" The service went long, over two hours, with loud, off-key hymns and hands waving wildly while the Scripture was read by a sweaty, red-faced man swaying over the pulpit.

Around the time it seemed like the service was ending, there was an announcement, and the pastor and my grandparents called me to the front of the small church with my family in tow. While we huddled on the small platform, the red-faced pastor spoke about my illness awkwardly, obviously uninformed, but he exchanged that lack of knowledge for fervor, spitting out words like, "Let us pray for God to heal her, release her, and unleash the illness from her young body!" I wore a red velvet dress that day and distinctly remember how its color brought out the discoloration on my arms and legs under the overhead church lights as I felt the eyes of strangers bore into my blotchy skin.

"Megan, get in the center here so we can all lay hands on you and pray," my grandpa said with an authoritative voice. What choice did I have, after all, as the congregation swarmed around us? My body was gently pushed toward the center of this hive, and amid a feeling of claustrophobia, my mind floated somewhere above us all, looking down as the scene unfolded. Hands on me—shoulders, arms, head—as mouths moved and words spilled out in passionate, indecipherable language. Toward the end of the prayer session, after the swarm of people returned to their seats, they asked me to remain.

"Megan, do you believe in God's healing?" my grandpa asked, eyes wide and hopeful.

My body was still stunned; I was on the spot and needed an answer that would remove me from this stage as quickly as possible. So I said yes, and with that, all the hands shot up even higher and feet stomped with excitement, making the chapel echo and shake. As I returned to my seat, attendees reached out to touch me as I passed by like I was some child celebrity.

We traveled home not long after that, but I still felt that congregation around me for months afterward, like an itchy turtleneck sweater that clung too tight yet was impossible to take off.

That next year, my scleroderma went into remission. It happened so quickly, disappearing as fast as the disease had initially occurred, that I felt confused. Had it ever existed at all? Was this all a strange dream? But no, the doctor's reports and imagery confirmed everything. The discoloration on my legs and arms faded, the shiny, scar-like tissue began to lighten, and I could wear a swimsuit without the smothering self-consciousness I'd felt before. However, that feeling lingered for years afterward, out of habit. I heard from my family that the people who had prayed for me at that mountain church all said it was a miracle, a gift from God as we gathered that day. Perhaps it was, or perhaps they needed it to be a miracle to confirm their ardent faith. Maybe it was a little of both: the prayers of others and the evolution of disease. No one can be entirely sure, but when I went back to the smelly doctor, he confirmed it was typical for scleroderma to go into remission on its own in children if they were diagnosed early enough.

This experience left me with a fascination around the body, like there is often something within us that lies deep beneath the surface if we dare to look. As I got older, I dove deep into studies of trauma and its residual impact on the body, and one day I found myself in a library where the books climbed high to the ceiling. One particular title grabbed my attention: *When the Body Says No* by Gabor Maté. I pulled the book from the shelf and opened it, and the very first words I read mentioned a client of his who was diagnosed with the same illness I had, albeit in adulthood. I was shocked. It was the first time I had read anything about scleroderma from a psychosomatic perspective. Before that, everything I'd read was clinical at best.

The first chapter opens with a story about a client who, from a young age, had learned to suppress her emotions, her voice, and her trauma to protect herself. It made Maté curious about the possible connection between her body's illness and that suppression. He wrote, "In scleroderma (from the Greek word meaning 'hardened skin'), the immune system's suicidal assault results in a stiffening of the skin."[1] He then asks two powerful questions: "Was scleroderma her body's way of rejecting this all-encompassing dutifulness?" and "What creates this civil war inside the body?"[2] His words offered a mirror to my experience I didn't even realize I needed at the time. There was something in me that longed to understand this disease and other illnesses my body held years later. Could they somehow represent the stories I carried inside and, possibly, the impact of repressing them?

I dug deeper into Maté's book—and later many others. He explained the disease's primary function was to create a thickening barrier through many layers of skin. *A civil war inside the body.* Yes, that was the language I had been searching for. There was a conflict under my skin, unspoken feelings and stories that lived in a fighting stance, impacting my immune system. Essentially, scleroderma is an autoimmune response that organizes an army, guarding from the inside out to protect the self from what the body interprets as a threat.

Learning all this got me thinking about the many ways I'd tried to protect myself over the years, emotionally and physically, and how I had learned to hide. I'd always struggled to share how I was feeling and about the sexual abuse that had shaped me as a young trauma survivor. This continued into adulthood with other experiences of sexual violence and assault that caused pervasive silence and overwhelming loneliness because I was never able to talk freely about my experience. I understand now that this is not uncommon. When our young selves experience painful events we are unable to contain, we create "safe houses" of our own construction to protect our stories and keep them locked away until we feel safe enough to open them. Perhaps that's what my body had been doing with this illness all along, trying to protect me from an internal war I had yet to name.

It is a thought I still sit with as I look at my skin while I type these pages: pale, thin, wrinkles beginning to form from the onset of middle age. Though this disease is no longer active on the surface of my body, except for some ambiguous scars that remain on my back, it will never entirely go away, a reminder of the hidden layers of story that lie dormant, waiting for me to call them to the surface as I become ready to know their origin.

Our skin, muscles, and organs store emotions that are repressed during trauma; our bodies can become holding cells for our anger, sadness, worry, and despair. "We are all living history books. Our bodies contain our histories—every chapter, line, and verse of every event and relationship in our lives," Caroline Myss explains. "As our lives unfold, our biological health becomes a living, breathing, biographical statement that conveys our strengths, weaknesses, hopes, and fears."[3]

The work I've discovered over the years is to understand that my body is not my enemy but instead my historian, my advocate, my storyteller, and my brilliant friend. She offers me gifts wrapped in skin and language, full of wisdom, waiting for me to open them. As poet Mary Oliver writes about being given "a box full of darkness," I, too, have come to understand that such a thing can indeed be a gift.[4] This reframe around the body can seem so contradictory. Still, when we approach the body's story with compassionate listening, we can heal our narrative one chapter at a time.

I have always been captivated by stories, stories both within and outside of me. I read anything I could get my hands on to connect with language, searching for words and experiences that mirrored my own. One of the first books that changed me was *I Know Why the Caged Bird Sings* by Dr. Maya Angelou. At twelve years old, I felt my hands shake as I read it. It was her telling of her childhood that gripped me the most, as she wrote about being a young trauma survivor and the muteness it created in her. I related to the unsayable she spoke of, the danger she must have felt within her own body from that hidden truth, obscured and floating. Never in my life had I experienced something so vulnerable. Her words became my lifeline, my Shawshank escape, my break out of this dark world, and, as the writer Franz Kafka wrote, "an axe for the frozen sea inside [me]."[5] It was as though Angelou gave me the permission I was looking for to uncover my truth, even if I didn't know what that truth was yet.

Many books that followed after Angelou served as a road map to discovering my love for stories—books from authors like Rumi, Khalil Gibran, Sheri Reynolds, Sylvia Plath, and so many more. These books mainly existed in the hallway of my childhood home on a wooden bookshelf that remains to this day a library stacked high, ranging through every genre imaginable. Books dog-eared and annotated, books started and left unfinished, books passed down from one generation to the next with dedications scribbled on the front page. It was a tradition; I assumed that after finishing one book I would go search those shelves for a new one my parents had just moved on from.

As I studied these authors' words, I wondered if I, too, could play with language and become a historian of my own lived experience. I began to test the theory, spilling my words out on paper until my soft fingers formed calluses, filling up pages with poetry and personal essays. It seemed that with every page I wrote, a light grew that exposed the ways I'd been hiding without realizing it, revealing a filter over my voice that had been silencing me mostly through emotional suppression, repressed trauma, and religious duty.

Like many growing up in the heart of the Bible Belt, I found religion to be a way of life, ritual, and identity. Before I ever entered a church building, God was in everything, every flower I smelled, every tree I climbed, and every lake I dipped my toes into. It seemed that in everything, God was befriending me. It was a welcome comfort to the sadness and secrets of trauma held in my young bones that made me ache without knowing why. After my skin disease diagnosis, a few years after my trip to my grandparents' church, I was desperately lonely and wanted to be part of something. All of my friends were going to church, getting saved, and singing in choirs, and so I decided to catch the same spiritual wave they were all riding.

At the time, this church setting offered relief from the inner ache I felt, but it also further exasperated the emotional suppression happening in my home life and the trauma repression that had been buried within my body. Still, I remained part of the church for years and integrated my identity so far into its theology that I couldn't tell the difference between who I was and what I was "supposed to be." It was impossible to name at the time, but I basically lost my voice and selfhood in the spiritual shuffle that went something like pray, repent, rinse, and repeat. As a result, I felt numbed out by the religious formula that served to inoculate me, like I was sleepwalking. The truth? I didn't want to feel anything, and there it was: a prescriptive numbness served free of charge on a communion platter that everyone else seemed to be partaking of. How could I refuse? I felt pain no one could see and that I couldn't quite identify.

I'd recognized this pain in Maya Angelou's memoir, which mirrored my silence and my feelings of stuckness and captivity. Her bird had finally broken free. Could mine? Her words made me feel less alone and taught me to bravely show up to the page in order to release the built-up emotions stockpiled in my body.

There was a question that became more pronounced with every word I wrote, a question that throbbed in my body: Was I ready to wake up and heal my life? If yes, then all signs pointed to a narrow path marked with all things dark and unknown. It terrified me and yet was the very thing I needed to face to feel alive: my sacred stories. Though by this time I had shifted away from the church as an institution, this journey into writing and creative expression through story healing brought me back to my faith in a new way. I learned the power of listening and having curiosity for the unanswered questions, and I found myself on an inner search that led me to deep spaces that scared me and yet, at other times, held me like a womb as I uncovered meaning for many unsayable moments of my life.

Annie Rogers, a psychoanalyst whose work has been so informative to my healing, writing, and research, wrote a book titled *The Unsayable: The Hidden Language of Trauma*.[6] This title rang true for me, and saying what had been unsayable became a foundational process in my journey toward using story healing as an act of revisiting my past stories in order to understand their impact on the past, present, and future through the act of writing and reflection. It became my life's expedition. I longed to understand the body as a storyteller and to use the power of writing to release my past pain. There was something about words that materialized what had felt stuck in my body when I read them and wrote them down.

As I began writing to heal my stories, especially the tender ones, it was as if the old trauma wounds began knocking at the door of my life, asking me to answer for the very first time. At first I resisted, fearing who I might find waiting for me on the other side. Still, as I began to ask what these stories wanted to show me, the door slowly opened, not with a bang but with a creaking, as if it was part of a haunted house waiting to be explored, a haunted house I wasn't necessarily afraid of but rather intrigued by.

The process of healing my stories has been painful but necessary, a process that continues to this day. Our stories are never done with us; they are constantly unraveling layer upon layer to help us create a deeper understanding of how to exist and be in this world.

In the book of Ezekiel, there is a story about a valley of dry bones. I've always likened this text to the trauma and pain held in our bodies—stories forgotten over time, left to dry out in the hot desert sun. We are told that when Ezekiel spoke words over those bones, they began to rattle and shake back to life, with skin, blood, and tissue clothing the bare skeletons until they were once again alive. Like those dry bones, trauma can remain dormant in us for years, until we give it language that helps it remember what it once was. When we listen to the stories within and put pen to paper, we are asking the same question of our lives: *Can these bones live?*[7] If we are still enough, we may see the stories rattle to life; we may hear them tell us mysteries of the past, and we may see a miracle.

Through this journey of healing my stories, I realized I wanted to help others do the same. But I didn't want to be a typical therapist. Instead, I craved a middle way between talk and somatic therapy. I wanted to be a story guide for those seeking to heal through writing and creative expression, to serve everyone who had a story waiting to be told and written. I earned my master's degree at a school that specialized in narrative-focused trauma care and spiritual direction, and during the program I dove into my own story by reflecting on the most formative moments in my life and researched the body as storyteller, learning how it becomes the gatekeeper for the stories too tender to address until we are emotionally available for them.

As I prepared to write this book, I thought of the many storytellers I've supported over the years and the themes that arose from our sessions that mirrored many of my own: origin stories that brought about self-doubt, overwhelm as it related to a need for control, the fear of truth-telling as it relates to parentification, and how the body contains unspoken narratives. I also thought about how important it is to include trauma-informed care in our story healing as it relates to the physiological fight, flight, freeze, or fawn response that can come with writing about past pain. After all, writing and trauma response relate to one another.

When we explore our stories with the tools of writing and the tools we need to heal our narratives, we can begin the work of rewriting the scripts that have shaped us over the years. But to begin even thinking about how we can use writing to heal, we must ask the question, To heal what? The stories we've bypassed over time because they've been forgotten or are too tender to confront. Why? To recover words lost to the unsayable in our bodies. How? Through creative expression and writing as a way to process past pain.

With all this said, I need to be clear. This is not a book just for writers and creatives. This is for every BODY who has experienced the good, the bad, and the ugly of life. There are stories within you waiting to be written and read because they will help you listen to and understand your life.

I'm not going to pretend this story healing isn't tender work, that it won't bring to the surface wounds you have left unattended for years or cause paper cuts from flipping through the many pages of your body's narrative as you search for truth. This journey is hard—but it is healing. Know this: if there is an aching in your life that needs healing, then beginning with writing your formative stories is a powerful portal to finding yourself. And no, you don't have to identify as a writer or creative to begin uncovering the power of your narrative. If you have a body, you have a story, a history, a manuscript made of the tissue, bone, and blood of a life lived.

Recently, a client asked me, "Will I feel better once I start writing down my stories?" I laughed. I didn't want to break her heart; she was so incredibly full of hope. "No," I said. "You will feel worse . . . at first." Her face fell. She wanted an easy answer, a quick fix, a shot of resolution I could not give her. The process of healing one's stories is a lifelong journey. Where one story begins, another one ends—all connected. We begin healing by examining the fabric of our lives, noting how one piece connects to another and another until it creates an entire quilt. Where there are holes in the fabric, I firmly believe there is also mending that comes when we make space to witness our truth, uncover our voice, and befriend the stories that live within us.

My hope for you, dear reader, is that this book awakens your stories, your healing journey, and your curiosity for writing and creative expression as tools for discovery. Throughout, I share vulnerable personal essays to illustrate story healing and therapeutic concepts. May they be a launching pad for your self-reflection and offer insight into how uncovering your stories, some broken into tiny pieces, can help make you whole once they are gathered together.

At the end of each chapter are writing prompts to help you begin examining your own story, along with affirmations you can repeat over yourself. These are not required for this reading, but they will help you dive deeply into your healing journey. I hope they serve you well as you write them down without apology or censure.

So here's the thing: Will this book bring up a lot for you? I hope so. I hope it disrupts you, shakes you, and makes you feel feelings you've forgotten about. I also hope it revives you. That it shines light on your hidden stories and forgotten wounds so that you can begin to heal them in the light of day.

PART 1
CHOICE

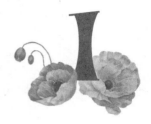

Collecting Memories

want to heal my stories, but where do I start?" It's one
of the first questions people ask me when they want to
dive into their story healing. They ask with voices shaking in longing and anticipation. I give the same answer every
time, without hesitation: start with your body, start with your
earliest memory, or, as Anne Lamott writes, "start with your
childhood."[1]

There are many ways to begin navigating the stories within,
but one of the ways I've spent my life exploring is through
writing and creative expression. Why? Because this is how
we begin to engage with the world from the beginning—our
little mouths mimicking sounds and language, our little ears
soaking up bedtime stories, our little fingers smearing paint
across paper, our little eyes taking in the contours of a person's
face to understand our own—all innate passages to knowing
ourselves and how we exist in the world.

When we're young, there is no "bad" way of learning to
speak, walk, draw a picture, or write a story. As cartoonist and

educator Lynda Barry writes, "How old do you have to be to make a bad drawing?"[2] Everyone knows it is just a beginning, a playground of becoming oneself without pretense. It's not until years later that art becomes subjective, and we forget the initial draw we felt to create in order to express ourselves. That's why healing our stories invites a return to that younger self to uncover our first moments and first memories that shape us so that we can touch on a foundation of truth that exists in its purest, most egoless form.

It is through collecting these earliest moments that we can begin to write a new story and reframe our past with compassion and care. So many stories have shaped us over the years, many of which we have never looked at in the light, though these same stories replay time and again in various ways—in our relationships, our creative direction, our belief or lack of belief in ourselves—when they are left unaddressed. This is why, sitting with these formative early moments, we can begin the process of rewriting and reauthoring our lives by constructing a new narrative. Not rewriting to change the story—wouldn't that be nice? Instead, writing as a way to reflect and find new meaning beyond our past pain.

When I started writing my earliest memories, I was searching for meaning in my own stories. This search was like diving deep into the ocean. The salt water burned my eyes and made my vision blurry, yet it was all worth it because I felt alive with wonder and curiosity for my life. Some of my recollections were filled with play and others were like hauntings—and both offered meaning and new understanding for who I was at my core.

"The first memory," psychoanalyst Alfred Adler writes, "will show the individual's fundamental view of life. I would never investigate a personality without asking for the first memory."[3] I resonated deeply with these words as I explored the complexity of memory. Early memories play an essential role in story healing, and we can use our first memory as a starting place in writing to know our truest selves. After all, the root meaning of *memory* is to commemorate, mourn, and visit a memorial to reflect on our lives. Remembering is a sacred act.

Whenever I propose using our first memories as a starting place, people ask, and rightfully so, "But what if I don't remember anything?" Their expression is locked in curiosity, and don't I know it? As a childhood trauma survivor, for me traversing memory as an adult has been like flipping through a book with torn-out pages. So when I speak of *memory*, believe me, I know the nuance, the shame, and the overwhelm at the very word in regard to writing and exploring stories of my past.

When I think about memory, I recall pink puffy clouds of fiberglass insulation. Growing up in the South, I saw it everywhere: in the open walls in my cousin's house, where it stuck through exposed wood planks, or when it was left abandoned on the side of a street after a big storm had come and leaked through the roof, turning it into a wet, purple mess. I knew it was bad for me, but sometimes I couldn't help but touch it, feel the fine prick of a thousand microneedles, and see the shards of fiberglass shine like glitter on my skin. Barely visible, that insulated memory of a life. The body knows, though, making these memories feel just as itchy as those fibers. Unseen from far away, up close they sparkle in the sunlight.

Years after my body began speaking, I heard it again in adulthood as prickles throughout my body from a nervous system shot after prolonged stress, a temporary disorder called *paresthesia*, which causes a person's skin to tingle and feel like pins and needles are under the surface of the skin. It felt just like touching that insulation. This disorder is common in those suffering from overwhelming stress and emotional dysregulation.[4] It made sense at the time. I was recovering from experiencing sexual assault in college, a traumatic experience I tucked away until the pinpricks became unbearable. My body was telling a story, and finally, with its persistent knocking, I became curious enough to begin paying attention.

A couple of years after the assault, the earthquake of my life had finally seemed to settle, and the only sound left was silence. Silence is louder than noise when you're not used to it. The years of stress, spiritual suppression, and trauma stories had created enough friction to shake my world up and bring on the tsunami of grief. An earthquake only ends when there is no energy left to sustain it. A tsunami only subsides when it exhausts itself on shore. In the same way, it was only when I'd finally wearied of playing hide-and-seek with my pain and decided to finally come up from the deep water that I could begin to interpret my stories, many of which looked like massive sinkholes seemingly impossible to fill or repair.

I don't say all this to dishearten but to highlight the realistic journey of writing through memory that is scattered. It is hard, but it is also transformational; it is, above all, a choice we must make every single day to listen to our lives and sit with them, even in their most dire hour. Think of it like this: when we do this story healing and dive into memory, we are acting as story doulas through the most beautiful and painful moments of recollection. As poet Joy Harjo writes so beautifully, we are to extend a welcome to our wandering spirits when they return, though "(they) may return in pieces, in tatters. Gather them together. They will be happy to be found after being lost for so long."[5]

So when I speak about memory, let me be clear: I am not talking about accuracy, something complete or perfectly whole. I am talking about gathering the scattered pieces of our stories and beginning to put them together. As Jodi Picoult describes it, "Memory is like plaster: peel it back and you just might find a completely different picture."[6] This is why when we start to write from our earliest memory, we must begin by listening to our bodies, our keepers of stories that existed before we had linear language—before our words formed a straight line of recollection rather than being crooked or altogether missing from our shattered memory.

As I explored the complexity of memory through writing, what I found shocking was not the pain from my more recent assault but rather echoes from childhood trauma left unaddressed. My search revealed debris piled high, the aftermath of many years of storm damage. It was my life—the good, the bad, the forgotten. Starting from the bottom, I began to sort through it all. One by one, I moved memories around like they were parts of a ten-thousand-piece puzzle, some pieces so old they crumpled on contact with the smell of wet mildew. Other memories were new, pristine, barely touched. Some larger pieces were easy to unpack; the small, fragmented ones were difficult to grasp, and some were missing altogether. But one memory at a time, I began to make sense of my life.

In order to help myself navigate through my memories, I decided to construct a timeline of my life so I could see a visual progression of my subconscious and conscious memories. First, along one side of the page, I wrote down all the ages, from zero to my current age. It was important that this timeline have very few rules; all I needed to do was select a word or short phrase for each age, using a timer, so that I could express myself without any measurement of right or wrong. Before I began, I took a deep breath and closed my eyes to picture the first word or visual that arose.

The next step, after forming my initial list, was to use each item as a prompt for further writing. Making this timeline was frustrating at first, as I found myself trying to tie memory to accuracy and only write what felt sensical, but when I reminded myself it was okay to let that go and trust my subconscious to guide the way, I was able to relax and find the words. From there, I gave myself a choice of which word to begin writing on and for how long.

This choice is essential. Memory work is tender work, so allowing ourselves the chance to choose where and how we begin is the key to feeling safe in the process. This took me some time to learn. At first, I would dive into writing the hardest memories without an ounce of precaution or the reminder that I could always choose to stop, take a break, or write on something different altogether. If I had held this reminder close from the beginning, it would have saved me a lot of unnecessary pain as I tried to rush through my healing. I implore you to let this choice be at the forefront of your process while creating your timeline. Writing from that place of choice will create a deep trust and agency in your story healing.

Before you begin, I also invite you to take a moment to consider how you can care for yourself in the process of creating your timeline. If you want to borrow my process, it was and continues to be incredibly simple: I set a timer for twenty minutes. I freewrite on the word I've chosen without judgment. I read it back to myself when I'm finished. Then I take a bath or shower as a symbol of washing myself clean from the past.

Here is a glimpse of what my initial timeline looked like:

Age 0: womb
Age 1: bathtub
Age 2: diaper
Age 3: bloody nose
Age 4: the bedroom wall

To an outsider, these words wouldn't make any sense. Honestly, at first glance they didn't make much sense to me either, but as I went through and wrote poems, stories, and visuals that arose based on each one, memories began to appear in a way that was surprising. It was as though they had been there all along but were far off and hard to see at a distance. I was discovering "islands in a sea of oblivion," as Esther Salaman writes in her book *A Collection of Moments.*[7] With this practice, I was stopping to visit each one of these memory islands with open eyes and an open heart.

Early memories that captured little moments like falling out of bed and getting a bloody nose, falling on the concrete in front of our house, or falling in a repeated dream—all of these made me curious about the theme of falling. One memory in particular stood out to me and compelled me to write about it. Here is what I wrote from my timeline for age four, the bedroom wall, based on one of my earliest memories:

My earliest memory exists between the wall and the side of my brother's bed, where I would fall into the narrow crack and cry out. Those late nights when the thunderstorms raged, and I swore the big trees would come crashing right down on me, I stumbled into my brother's bedroom and crawled into his tiny twin bed where it was safe and warm. Then, at some point after the storm cleared and there was only the ceiling fan circling above, I would wake with a claustrophobic feeling of stuckness, my little body wedged somewhere it was never meant to be—collapsed between mattress and wall.

This is not a metaphor. This is not some way to hint at dreams, trauma, or some other something that could be threaded from this description. No, this is the imagery I return to whenever someone says, tell me about your earliest memory. I see the pasty white wall inches from my face. I feel the cotton mattress against my back. I hear the soft breathing of a brother. I smell the musty attic and old, thick carpet. I taste the salty tears ballooning in the back of my throat before they release. I believe I cried out, and someone came and pulled me out of the stuck place, but no one can be sure now. That's not really the point anyway. The point is that our earliest memory asks us: Do you want to be awake to your stories? Do you want to heal through the process of listening to what's within you?

When I sit with this writing—the details, the imagery, the effect—the themes of this memory rise to the surface: loneliness, falling, fear, silence, and stuckness. These same themes show up when I break down the most defining moments of my life: the *loneliness* in my relationships, even within the safety and love of my decade-long marriage; the *falling* effect in my emotional windfalls, so severe I felt dizzy; the *fear* in recalling my trauma narratives that were located far into the past, yet when spoken about felt closer than ever before; learning to *silence* my voice at home and in religious settings so as to not rock the boat; and the *stuckness* that showed up in my writing as a sort of creative block. These five words thematically represent my earliest memory in my waking life. In recognizing these themes, I have been able to make connections when they show up in my life time and again. There is no longer surprise, disdain, or frustration at the arrival of these themes, now that I know them, just a recognition. *I see you. I know why you're here. Have a seat; I've got this now.* This knowledge allows me to take the driver's seat of my stories rather than just watch those old themes from my past play out.

After I began working on this timeline and memory excavation, I also learned so much about the importance of taking my time and not rushing this process. Each memory held an important meaning and sometimes was emotionally difficult to process. I listened to my body and wrote only one memory a week, then processed it with my therapist and close friends. This was a powerful act because not only did it bring that moment out of the shadows but it also welcomed other trusted people into my inner world to help me decipher meaning.

If I were to ask you to tell me about your earliest memory, what would come to mind? Again, this is not about factual accuracy. This is about becoming curious about the stories within you, listening to them with an open heart, and releasing them without judgment onto the page to reflect on as a compassionate witness of your life.

One important truth that has given me hope around these "holey" memories (see what I did there?) is realizing that these memory gaps serve us for a reason. Maybe the experiences that have gone missing were too painful for us to reconcile at the time, and so the body and brain did what they needed to do to protect us from them. Whatever the case, memories, whether lost or found, exist first and foremost in our bodies, even if we can't consciously recall them.

When you think about the importance of healing your stories and where to start, close your eyes and lean into that earliest memory. What does your body tell you? What do your senses say? What visual comes to mind? What emotional truth? Our bodies are libraries. They know the stories we avoid telling because they are so damn real—but often the ones the world needs most.

WRITE ON THIS:

Create a Timeline

I know how scary it can be to return to those early memories, especially when our memories feel like missing puzzle pieces.

   This is why I invite you to create a timeline of your life to dig into your subconscious body memory. Again, this is not about writing logically or with accuracy but with your intuition.

   Begin by listing each age, from zero to your current age. Next to each number, write the first word, phrase, or visual that comes to mind. Don't question its absurdity; trust that your subconscious is speaking.

   After creating this timeline, pick one age to write about (ideally before age ten). Write a short story or poem based on that age and the word associated with it, starting with this line: My earliest memory begins with . . .

REPEAT AFTER ME

*My memory is a doorway
for healing and recovery.*

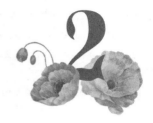

The Power
of Genesis Stories

When I think of beginnings, I am ushered back to memories of the first day of school, with its hour-long indecision of what I could wear that would be deemed "cool enough," only to discover that the new shoes I thought were in style were totally outdated; the social anxiety that knotted my stomach thirty minutes before the first bell rang, causing me to hunker down in the bathroom stall, a welcome hiding place from the bustle of a new classroom; how I'd ask my mom to drop me off a block away from the school entrance, then watch her drive away so I could skip class and walk the long mile back home to watch *Days of Our Lives* and eat Hot Pockets.

Beginnings have always been a source of stage fright for me, be it a new class, a new relationship, or a new project. This fear is also at the beginning of healing our stories. Just as endings involve a journey through a grieving process that includes acknowledging the emotional upheaval, beginnings have a similar journey—through our fears rather than around them. This can only happen when we are willing to choose the risk of staying put when everything inside us wants to run away.

Usually, this fear of beginning stems from origin stories that are keeping us attached to old fears. Stories that shape our self-worth, our ability to trust others, and our confidence in our own voices. There are so many messages we grow up with that are implanted in our psyche from a young age. Messages from friends, family, teachers, mentors, the environments around us. These voices can be both positive and negative, but often the negative messages are the ones we cling to the hardest.

Think about it—you get ten compliments and one critique that says you could do better. What do you focus on? The one critique, right? I totally get it, and so do most people. According to neuroscientific evidence, the brain has a stronger response to negative stimuli, often referred to as a "negativity bias,"[1] that has been ingrained in us from early development, affecting how we see, experience, and take risks in the world and in relationships.

Before I began digging into my stories, those old voices showed up often with megaphones that boomed. I tried to ignore them, but that only seemed to make them louder. I would hear these voices anytime I took a risk by making a vulnerable attempt to tell my stories. *That's not going to be good enough; what makes you so special? Do you think you have something unique to share?* Even as I write about it now, I remember how those voices felt, so thick and omniscient.

When I finally learned about origin stories—the defining moments of our past, the stories that form us from a young age and shape our belief systems—it gave those old voices context. It was apparent I could no longer run from them, so I had a choice: I could begin to name them, or I could just learn how to better manage their ongoing chatter in my head. I chose the former. I knew there were things beneath the surface of these stories that, if I could name them, would allow me to lay them to rest. This naming hasn't made them disappear entirely, but they no longer dominate my life. When these old voices make themselves known today, I set my boundaries, let myself feel as I need to, and keep moving forward with the reminder that as I pay attention to these old stories rather than ignore them, I can continue to edit a past that was formative but no longer defines me.

I've started calling these origin stories "Genesis stories," since they relate to the beginning of our earliest moments— when we went from nothing to something, a living, breathing, embodied story. After all, I grew up on the book of Genesis, fed from a young age by Bible stories my grandma would read to me as she tucked me in at night. One of my favorites was the first chapter of Genesis, probably because it was filled with animals and the ocean, both of which I loved (and still do today) but also because it spoke to the heart of storytelling and creation.

The book of Genesis begins with the line, "In the beginning . . . the earth was without form, and void; and darkness was on the face of the deep."[2] My grandma would read me this passage with wild hand gestures and whooshing sounds, making the water come alive. When she described it I felt as if I could see the ocean's darkness, the bigness of everything in creation—both mesmerizing and terrifying.

This passage comes back to me whenever I am unraveling a new story, a vast landscape asking me to explore it. I see the blank canvas awaiting the splattering of paint, the blank screen with its blinking cursor awaiting words, the blank journal page awaiting spilled ink from unprocessed freewriting—all waiting to be created upon. I think about those Genesis words and how they reveal the bigness of beginnings and the fears that threaten to capsize so many of us when we begin writing our stories and releasing them from our bodies.

Whenever I talk with someone about what is holding them back from writing their personal stories, usually the first thing they say is, "I just feel overwhelmed by beginning at all." That is when I ask them to describe this overwhelm, the texture of it, to give their fear of beginning a name—and guess what the majority of them call it?

The void.

The void is the blankness that covers the surface of the deep, the empty pages. It echoes our fear of the unknown and our inability to predict what will be created. To use the image from Genesis 1, these origins are *without form*, shapeless putty in the hand of an artist that must be formed to become anything at all. By necessity we live out our lives as the sacred first drafts that we are, messy and full of stories.

There is also *the darkness* that hovers over the pulse of a project—the self-doubt that arises when we dare to begin to let the pen hover over the pages of our lives with the chance to make beauty and/or disaster.

To address the beginnings that stall us and to face off with the void, we must consider our own stories of beginning: how they've shaped us, inspired us, and terrified us. We must practice releasing our attachment to those Genesis stories by acknowledging the past. Author Sarah Manguso states it so beautifully in her book *Ongoingness*: "Perhaps all anxiety might derive from a fixation of moments—an inability to accept life as ongoing."[3] In other words, we must name our fear of confronting these Genesis stories so that we are not controlled by them.

It wasn't until I was in my twenties that I began to address my own need for control, a compulsion that extended from my childhood trauma. I'd even invented a game called Worst-Case Scenario, which I would "play" by listing every possible outcome that could happen to avoid surprises. I desperately needed to prevent the shock of the unknown from being able to derail me.

One day, while I was with my therapist, I thought back to being in my childhood bedroom, creating an escape plan for any intrusion that *might* occur. Before going to sleep, I would pick the most accessible hiding spots so that if I heard a scary sound or sensed a threat, I'd know exactly where to run. I had three go-to escape options: my dirty laundry basket, which I could crawl inside and then pile clothes on top of my little body (this one was my favorite); behind my mattress bedframe because under the bed would be way too obvious (hello, every scary movie ever made); and lastly, the far back corner of my bedroom closet, which I kept as an empty space for me to fit into if the occasion called for it. To my recollection, I never needed to use any of these hiding places, but the ability to predict and control helped me feel safe.

It wasn't until I was recounting this practice of ritualistic protection that my therapist confirmed that this is not what most kids who felt safe did. "They don't?" I asked, my eyes wide in surprise.

I had no idea—yet there I was, repeating the same game decades later in her office. My eyes scanned the room, looking for any cues about what might happen or be said next. My restless legs shook at an impossible speed, making the floor tremble until it felt like a minor earthquake. I even faced the exit so I could remind myself there was a quick way out if I needed it (something I still do today out of habit).

I listened as she introduced me to the language of "hyper-vigilance as a trauma response," which my therapist defined as being on high alert to any potential threat or danger. This hyper-vigilant response was innate and something my body needed to do to feel safe and in control of my environment. When I began to work with the hypervigilance that had been conditioned in my nervous system as a way to predict my world, I started with learning to recognize why it existed in me in the first place. I was a child whose story and emotional truth had been displaced and unnamed, so I created safety mechanisms to feel supported, even if those mechanisms turned compulsive over the years.

When I began to heal my stories, I knew that to get to the heart of them, I needed to start releasing my grip on control in order to begin the process of naming how I felt, the experiences that impacted me, and the ways I participated in my own hide-and-seek games. Games that even showed themselves in my story work as a college student, when I would write essays on my family of origin to which my professor responded with the comment, "Must I go search for you in every sentence?" He was right; I was hiding even behind language, ducking behind one metaphor after another.

Over time, I began to come out of hiding the more I practiced naming the feelings and experiences that shaped me. I also renamed my experiences with greater compassion and empowerment as someone who had lived through to the other side of them. In narrative therapy, this is known as reauthoring or re-storying.[4] People are encouraged to think deeply about their lives and uncover new meaning beyond the prescribed narratives handed them. Narratives that perpetuate a family dynamic, a role in a relationship, or a belief in oneself that keeps them stuck in the same cycle.

I needed to name my need for control and how the hypervigilance in my body helped me feel contained, and there are many other ways that naming and renaming can support those becoming awake to their Genesis stories for the first time. Think about it like this: a person begins to say they were a sensitive child growing up and were emotionally reactive to everything. Their renaming of that experience will grant them a deeper understanding of why: They were a sensitive child because their emotionally volatile home environment meant they had to learn to read the room at a young age. That emotional attunement, which they once observed as a weakness, they now understand to be a superpower that allowed them to feel safe.

Another person may feel the compulsion to keep their house so clean that there is never one spot of dust or a chair pushed out of place. They are called a neat freak and feel embarrassed by their need to fix things. They begin to say that they feel really stressed when things are out of order and feel at peace when they can clean or put something back into place. Their renaming takes this further: They were a child in an abusive home in which the abuse was triggered by any spill or mess that was made. They learned to preemptively keep everything clean to avoid violence, a behavior that persists even decades later. This re-storying allows them to say, "I found safety in keeping things in order because it wasn't safe to be messy and playful as a child. Now, I can bless the parts of me that need structure and see that my actions are an act of protection for my younger self."

Both these examples are of people who have chosen to name something true within themselves so that they can begin to rewrite their stories. Another key to this process is understanding that these Genesis stories often highlight only a fraction of a lived experience instead of the multitude that creates the complete whole.

Not long ago, I watched a TED Talk with novelist Chimamanda Adichie called "The Danger of a Single Story" in which she articulates the problematic nature of leaving many facets of a story unnamed or only being aware of a single narrative. Growing up in Nigeria, she had been exposed to only a single side of a story in American and British books that left out women like her. Not only that, but when women of color were included, it was in a discriminatory and stereotypical light. Ultimately, she was unable to find herself on the pages of these one-sided narratives, and in her TED Talk she described the devastating implications incomplete stories and erasure of another's experience can have. Adichie shares, "The single story creates stereotypes, and the problem with stereotypes is not that they aren't true but [that] they are incomplete. They make one story become the only story."[5]

This is why story healing is akin to an awakening. It invites us to pay attention to our lives, to stay awake to our inner and outer worlds, and to chase with a fury the questions that arise from our Genesis stories. The questions, not necessarily the answers, are the pulse of healing our stories. As poet Rainer Maria Rilke wrote, "Do not now seek the answers, which cannot be given to you because you would not be able to live them. . . . *Live* the questions now. Perhaps you will then gradually . . . live along some distant day into the answer."[6]

And so, this is how we begin to name our Genesis stories: we step back. We step back to face the past in order to step forward. We pay attention. We dive into the void, the formless unknown, the darkness. We write from the scary places we avoid most, and we watch ourselves survive as we do it again and again, each time with a little more curiosity, self-kindness, safety, and choice in how we approach the stories of our lives along the way.

WRITE ON THIS:

Genesis Stories

We all have Genesis stories that shape us growing up. When we see these beginning moments as fundamental to how we experience the world, then we can have more understanding to choose how we respond to our old fears that arise in the form of past narratives. Ultimately, we can name the monsters we've been scared of. When exposed to the light, they don't look so big.

It is empowering to realize that we are not just being ushered along in the narrative of life but are actively involved with the process of how we tell our stories. What comes to mind when you think about the importance of naming and renaming your stories? Is there a particular story you have been gripping that is asking you to finally release it? How would your understanding of the story change as you begin to re-story yourself?

If you could give your life chapter titles, what would they be? Create a table of contents for your overall life story with twelve distinct chapter titles that summarize the evolution of what you've learned and uncovered over the years.

REPEAT AFTER ME

*I am not controlled
by narratives of my past;
I am rewriting my future.*

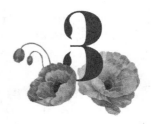

This Is for the Truth-Teller

When I began to write, remember, and own my truth, I was almost thirty years old. I learned at a young age that people felt better when I felt better, so I began to take on roles that people around me needed. This is not uncommon, especially for those who have experienced early trauma and take precautions that allow them to feel safe. There are so many of us who, later in life, feel a sense of identity theft as we begin to name the many roles we have played and the ways we have kept silent in the name of being safe. We put these roles on like an outfit, often forgetting to take them off even years or decades later because we are so used to them.

Family systems theory highlights at least five common roles: the golden child, the scapegoat, the mascot, the lost child, and the caretaker.[1] The golden child is the perfect one who can do no wrong. The scapegoat typically holds the focus of the family problems. They might also be known as the black sheep or the one who went their own way. The mascot absorbs the conflict in the family, often distracting away tension with a performance or a smile. The lost child tries to exist outside of the limelight to avoid blame or disappointment, usually feeling invisible as a result. Lastly, the caretaker takes on the responsibility of being the fixer or family therapist, all while neglecting their own needs.

I've played many of these roles over time; maybe you have too. When I began my story healing and began supporting others in uncovering their own stories, I saw these roles begin to break apart as I told the truth so that I could see the most authentic version of myself.

One of the roles I often took on was as an emotional caretaker, with the empathic ability to read the moods of others and try to soothe them. In psychology the word for this is *enmeshment*, a concept introduced by family therapy pioneer Salvador Minuchin to describe families in which personal boundaries are diffused and overconcern for others leads to a loss of autonomous development.[2] This usually comes to be either through family patterns passed unwittingly down from one generation to the next or through some sort of early trauma. A child growing up in an enmeshed home struggles to discern how to set boundaries, feels responsible for others' well-being, and avoids conflict at all costs by avoiding the word *no* in order to stay in others' good graces. A necessary process called *individuation* must take place in order for the child to identify as a separate self, but those who struggle to grab hold of that autonomy can remain stuck in this loop of enmeshment with family and in codependent relationships with others.

In assuming a caretaker role, I became a boundaryless kid who craved to live her truth but had no idea how. Somewhere along the way, I learned that I was really good at dissolving the sadness, anger, and overwhelm of others with scripted actions that played on repeat: *Do you feel sad and need me to compose a joyful monologue to distract you? Are you stressed out? I can put on a calming voice. Or perhaps you feel desperately lonely? I can act out an intimate persona that fills your ache for a short time.* It seemed I had a natural gift for creating an air of ease where there was exaggerated tension. No instruction manual taught me this. Instead, it was a learned behavior that came through adapting to others' needs, offering me the camou- flaged hiding place I needed and the approval and safety I was searching for when it felt impossible to be myself. Peter Levine, a somatic psychologist, describes it well: "When chil- dren are asked to 'turn the other cheek,' 'put on a happy face,' or 'strike back' in situations where they are experiencing daily terror, they do not learn character. On the contrary, they lose self-confidence and a sense of safety necessary to succeed."[3] I acted this way because it made life seem easier and lighter for everyone around me—and, if I'm honest, myself as well because I couldn't bear the weight of disappointing those I loved. Yet every time I sacrificed some part of myself in this way, I felt like I disappeared a little bit more.

No one told me to lie. No one said, *Just be happy, get it to- gether, put a smile on your face.* At least, not that I remember. It was just a daily hard pill I swallowed in order to navigate the environments I occupied as a young woman, as part of a fun- damentalist Christian church, and as part of a Southern meth- odology. Each one seemed to advertise a "put-togetherness" that I couldn't access internally but could project to the outside world.

Through these enmeshed and boundaryless environments, I became a master at putting a smile on my face and praying the bad away—but at the cost of my inner world splitting. It is a hard thing to live caught between the truth and a lie, but you can do it if you turn your back on the parts of yourself that are hard to embrace. And so that's what I did; I began to lie the way kids lie. Little fibs to assuage moments of potential disruption.

Soon, the practice became a habit, and after a while, I couldn't even tell when I was doing it anymore.

I can't tell you when it started because I was so young, but I had an unconscious reflex to lie whenever there was an opportunity to share my truth. These lies showed up often and in utterly casual ways, like in the days of high school when I would lie in bed well after my morning alarm went off. My mom would enter my room and press a hand to my forehead to feel my temperature.

"Are you feeling sick?" she'd ask.

I'd sputter a soft cough even though there was nothing wrong with my lungs or chest. "Yeah, I don't feel good. I need to stay home." Then I'd stare at her long and hard to see if she would catch the lie. The honest answer—the truth—if I dared to say it was, "No, I'm not sick. But I am scared to go to school." Yet I could find no words to explain how the intensity of my social anxiety made me hurl every day before first period.

There were other questions my college roommates would ask when I'd be in my room for days on end. "Hey, Megan, are you okay?" A thoughtful question but an anemic one, too broad for me to find an answer to. Instead of explaining my sadness, I'd usually respond with some paper-thin lie: "I'm totally fine, just tired." In truth, I had no words that could explain the depression that sucked my joy dry when I could hear their laughter that came so easily from the other side of the dorm room wall. These little lies just felt easier—until they didn't anymore. Over time, the truth began to stack up in my body. I was running out of room and had to make a choice: either start telling the truth to myself and others or fully embrace the roles that hid the true me.

There were several pivotal moments when I took the risk to share my truth, but the first one that stands out to me took place at a Chili's. You know—the all-American chain restaurant with the big red pepper on the front of the building. It was the go-to place for me and my friends in our late teens. The crowded booths filled with families, the smell of sizzling fajitas in the air, and the largest menus you've ever seen, second only to the Cheesecake Factory. I'm not kidding; a single menu would nearly take over the entire tabletop when opened up.

On this rainy day, I sat across the table from a family member as we sipped on sodas and dipped our tortilla chips in the never-ending bowl of salsa. I had decided to finally gather up the courage to share that I had been sexually abused, in, yes, the most casual and colorful ambiance ever, an environment that was the antithesis of my story. After I told them, there was a long pause. Then they asked, "Are you sure that's what really happened?"

This was not a response I had anticipated. The question hit me from across the table like a hard slap. They casually dipped their chip deeper into the salsa bowl as the waitress walked by and refilled our glasses. My words felt small as I stared across the table into their eyes, which now felt farther away than when we first arrived.

"Yes, I'm sure," I said quietly.

But as I said it, I suddenly wasn't so sure anymore. The restaurant's mood heightened with bustling servers and casual laughter that roared from a few tables over. My body felt hot with the shame of sharing, sweating through my clothes despite the ice-cold air-conditioning. The conversation dissolved quickly after that. I slipped into a more accommodating role by sharing a joke to jump off this train wreck of truth I'd attempted before it derailed into something even more shameful.

There are some words that have the ability to invalidate someone's experience so completely. Those six ordinary words, "Are you sure that really happened?" had the power to erase my lived experience, the memory I had of my past, and the courage it took to speak all of this in my own voice.

Yet even though this experience of truth-telling was heartbreaking, there was also empowerment in choosing to tell the truth. It was a starting place for me, a launchpad for trusting myself to share a story with boldness and zero apologies. However, in the future, maybe not at a Chili's and maybe not with a person who, at the time, could not hear me in the first place.

The second pivotal moment in speaking my truth came years after this Chili's incident when I said no to my parents for what felt like it was the first time ever. I was practicing saying no as a complete sentence, as author Anne Lamott writes,[4] by setting a boundary I never had before with, well, anyone.

I was in therapy for the first time, learning to acknowledge a codependency with my family so intense that when I was invited to step away from them in order to step forward into autonomy, I feared something might break. Their hearts? Their approval of me? The "good girl" rules I had adopted in that emotional caretaker role? I wasn't sure, but the fear of what might shatter was so prevalent I froze at the thought of it.

It had only been a year since I'd moved away from home when my parents said they wanted to visit me that summer in the beautiful Pacific Northwest. However, I wasn't emotionally ready to see them yet. I was just beginning to live without the enmeshed roles I'd assumed for so long. Doing so made me feel completely naked, and who goes to a nude beach with their parents? Not this lady. This brand-new boundaried autonomy I was practicing felt utterly fragile, too fragile to take on the challenge of seeing them. I felt a deep sense that I should protect my infant autonomy and set this essential boundary for the sake of my selfhood, which I was just beginning to define though I was in my late twenties. So I told them no when they asked to come see me. My mother cried, my body shook in fear of their disappointment, and I hid in my apartment that beautiful summer.

I said no that day, a word so small and yet so colossal in its impact that it felt like the world might just split in two at my parents' disapproval. You see, ever since I was young, this feeling of shame was the thing I was most afraid of. Disappointing someone you love is a bitter pill to swallow. But I had to say no. It was a word I needed to own. I had sacrificed so much for everyone else's yesses over the years. There, in that terrifying moment, it was time to take back my voice, even if doing so collapsed the good girl illusion I had perpetuated for years. Holly Whitaker describes this well:

> Saying no to people who want you to say yes, and upholding your boundaries with people who were used to you having none, will at first feel terrible, like death, and it is a death of sorts—the death of the part of you that thinks you have to violate yourself to make it in life or be valued.[5]

Speaking that one word made me feel the earthquake of family disruption; I shook violently for months. I want to tell you that I felt so empowered right after that moment of saying no, but instead I felt traumatized by my own boldness. The truth is everything I feared most about saying that word *did* happen—the disappointment, the disapproval, the separation, the shame. Still, once I made it through the rupture, repair could finally begin within myself, with my family, and with others close to me, this time with my autonomy intact. Though setting this boundary felt like a foundation was breaking and there was no one to prevent the collapse, I survived. Not only that, but I crawled out of the rubble more embodied, believing in myself, and with a deeper understanding of the roles I'd taken on at a young age and the enmeshed environments that had stalled out my emotional development. Saying no to my parents was an essential boundary that brought about growing pains in adulthood so that I could begin to trust myself and my family in a more holistic and true way.

This practice of saying no helped me stand my ground and empowered me in ways I'd never experienced. It seemed to say to me, *Megan, you can speak your truth, you can disappoint others, you can feel the shame, and after all of it, you will survive.* This was life-changing. When I'd said no before, it had felt like giving myself a death sentence; now, with this word, I felt more alive than ever. The death I'd feared most by voicing my need was actually the death of a persona, an expectation, a duty I'd fulfilled, a commandment written on a stone that I now boldly broke to pieces for the sake of my selfhood. I could finally grieve those old roles I used to play so that I could begin to live into something more authentic, more me.

To heal our stories, tell our truth, and write from the hard places, we must be willing to confront the past. Our past is here in the present, whether we want to admit to it or not. If we haven't addressed a rejection from an old friend, then we will keep replaying it with every new friend we make until we do. The same goes for our romantic relationships or our father-, mother-, sister-, or brother-wounds. If we have yet to work through our feelings of shame with those close to us, then we will continue to rehearse the shame cycle in our future relationships, seeking to heal a relational wound but without the proper medicine.

One shame cycle I stayed in was with my husband, Landon, early in our relationship, playing out the same wounded dynamics that I'd left unaddressed, like fear of vulnerability or early codependence. I nearly sabotaged our budding connection. But as I grew more and more aware of what was taking place and received his steady care, and as I evolved into more of me, the foundation of our relationship was grounded more securely in the truth I was beginning to name in myself, and him in his.

Being a truth-teller is not easy; it can be incredibly painful. But when we own our voices as truth-tellers, it can be life-altering. This work of using our voices is a muscle we must train, and it becomes stronger each time we do it—in speaking, in writing, and in saying no.

Know this: a truth-teller is a healer, a rebel, a disrupter, and a catalyst for change. A truth-teller shakes us to our core, makes us honest, confronts our demons, and validates our desires. A truth-teller is a spiritual guide, an artist, and a word warrior. A truth-teller is a sword that divides us and a healing balm that unites us. A truth-teller is wild and dangerous and the liberator we need. A truth-teller is not an identity we arrive at but a choice we make every single day when we advocate for our own voices. So speak your truth, feel the fear, and be the truth-teller you long to be because you are worthy of it.

WRITE ON THIS:

Truth-Teller Manifesto

We have all played roles in our families, work, and relationships. The roles we assumed when we were younger tend to be played out into adulthood, especially if we don't recognize how and why they exist in the first place. Were you ever the golden child, the scapegoat, the mascot, the lost child, or the caretaker? When you think back on the most dominant role you've played in your family, what was it? Does that same role show up when you are writing a personal narrative?

After reflecting on these questions, write your own Truth-Teller Manifesto on what that role means to you, beginning with these words: *A truth-teller is . . .*

Put your manifesto somewhere close by so you can return to it often.

REPEAT AFTER ME

I am a truth-teller with a story that's meant to be heard.

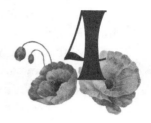

You Are the Gatekeeper

There's a picture of six-year-old me with my four-year-old cousin. We're wearing my dad's guitar, having loosened the strap to fit it over both our shoulders, and are dressed identically in oversized button-up shirts that hung down to our ankles and loose neckties that dangled down our centers, smiling wide with black mustaches drawn with my momma's mascara. I remember that moment well. During a party at my house filled with family and friends to entertain, I sought to remedy any chance of awkward silence and grabbed my little cousin, whom I employed, often against her will, to stand on the social stage of my own making. We burst into the living room, singing loudly and strumming the guitar so hard the strings nearly broke. The audience laughed, and we took bows, big and brave, as if we were on a New York stage.

As a kid, I loved the spotlight and ached for it, jumping in front of cameras with a desperate cry for attention. "Over here! Over here!" I'd yell and wave frantically until someone saw me and pressed record. But something changed when I finally got my chance to perform for real. I wasn't just excited; I was terrified. I was in fourth grade, performing a solo for the first time. The stage was dark except for the spotlight that hit me, so bright it made spots in my eyes. The piano notes began but I froze, words escaping me like a runaway horse. The notes came around again, cycle after cycle, until finally, the spotlight became less bright, and I could see soft eyes in the audience waiting for my voice to break through. To my right, my music teacher whispered the lyrics; I closed my eyes, took a deep breath, and let the song pour from my trembling mouth in a shaky vibrato.

Even though putting myself out there for all to see terrified me, I still craved the spotlight. No matter how many times people said, "The more you do it, the less afraid you'll be," I never knew this phrase to be true. If anything, the more I performed, the more I anticipated the shaking that would come from making myself vulnerable. In other words, I was shaking from the shaking.

There was this felt sense of being "too much" as I stood in the spotlight with my wild pursuit of attention. And yet, paradoxically, it never felt like I was enough to satiate the crowd, to please people. This feeling of "too much / not enough" has lived within me since I was that young performer, but it became pronounced as I wrote stories about my life. I found myself shaking there, too, a feeling strangely familiar to stage fright.

"Am I too much?"

To this day, that is one of the most common questions I receive from people writing about their lives. They hand over their stories to me, their truth dripping from the pages, and there, in the margins, I see this question highlighted for me to respond to: "Is it too much?"

It is a question I am repeatedly asked in my work as a writing coach as well as one I know well in my own life. A question I have been asking myself since I was young. A question that is less about writing and more about whether we have permission to be emotional, soulful, living, and loud truth-telling people.

Am I too much? I see little me jumping into the spotlight and jumping in front of video cameras, seeking attention anywhere I could get it, so insatiable for the praise of others and yet so terrified of the "too muchness" that came along with having a personality so *full*.

"Calm down, Megan."

"Choose to focus on one thing, Megan."

"You're so sensitive, Megan."

"Don't be so serious, Megan."

"Be happy again, Megan."

And on it went . . . a spiral of who I was and yet who I was not fully supposed to be. Too much / not enough.

Another version of "Am I too much?" rose in me on the cusp of pre-adolescence, when I became so aware of my body and wondered what others thought of me, the wild wave of hormones crashing through me without any understanding why. For children, such language is nowhere to be found. There is no sense that our first attempt at singing is bad or that we need to give up that silly dream of being an artist. No, we take up space in the rooms we occupy, paint pictures and think they're masterpieces, and tell everyone our dreams of being exactly what we want to be. We don't question it, at least not until someone tells us it's "too much."

Growing up as the youngest with two older brothers, I was a hybrid kid—a girly girl who played with Barbies and offered motherly advice to my dolls in need but was also half-tomboy, climbing to the tops of magnolia trees and catching minnows at the nearby duck pond. When my older brother was left to babysit me, much to his disdain, I would follow him around, mimicking his movements and style in desperate attempts to be "cool" just like him. All the while, he would shake me off as an annoying little sister who clung too close. He and his friends had a confidence that I craved and couldn't quite grasp. It was apparent to me that "boys" just seemed to know something I didn't, some inside secret that existed in being a young male in society, an innate sense of "enoughness" that I wasn't sure existed for me in all my girlness.

I felt this same feeling in church settings years later when I watched the boys serve communion at altars while the girls only partook of it, and the young men led music while the young women only sang soft harmonies in the background. Older men served as pastors, preaching from the pulpit, while the women—the wives—only sat taking notes fervently from the pews. Once again, the males seemed to know something, have something, that we females just couldn't quite grasp—a right to lead, to shepherd, to speak while we watched in quiet obedience.

I was well into adulthood when I began asking hard questions about my stories and using writing as a way to understand my life. I noticed I was playing this narrow role even within the pages of my own self-expression. I tried to write vulnerable stories without a filter but then questioned whether it was "too much," and I held back from being truly honest with myself.

On the page, the safest place I knew, I began to feel claustrophobic, caught between two walls of expectation closing in on me—"too much" and "not enough." How many of us have minimized our stories, passions, and emotions to be more palatable to those unable to receive what they haven't confronted in themselves? The anger, the sadness, the long-ing, the unrepressed expression, the unapologetic ache for something more—the raw truth.

When I started to help folks dive into writing their stories, I noticed that the women I worked with would begin writing truthfully until the question "Is it too much?" stopped them in their tracks. They asked it with concern and fear about their honesty, often feeling the need to erase their words even before finishing a complete thought. I also worked with men, yet in every single session I had with men writing about their lives, this question of "Is it too much?" never surfaced in our time together. NOT ONCE.

Thinking about the difference between these experiences, I couldn't help but wonder if this question was formed from the patriarchal society in which so many of us have grown up. A conditioned system that measures how women "should" behave. A system that tells women to speak up, but not too loudly. Serve others, but don't be a pushover. Be a leader, but don't be bossy. At what point do young girls go from believ-ing in their significance to doubting their stories matter? Is it a single moment or many compounded one after another, cemented by the patriarchal message we're indoctrinated with from a young age that corrupts our longing to understand and tell our stories? This is a nuanced conversation that often misses including other voices who have been impacted by this system, such as people of color, those with disabled bodies, and LGBTQ persons.

At the heart of this conversation around "Am I too much / not enough?" is really the topic of gatekeeping. As it sounds, *gatekeeping* implies controlling access, be it to a place, a per-son, or a story. When we think about the process of healing and writing our stories, we must be willing to look at who have been our gatekeepers in the past and perhaps even in the present. If you picture the moments in your life that have shaped how you view yourself as "too much" or "not enough," who is at the front of those stories? Perhaps it's a teacher who said you were underperforming, a jealous friend who said you were just trying to get attention, a family member who said you were too sensitive, or a religious leader who said you should be submissive toward authority. There are so many more we can name, but each of these is a shining example of a story gatekeeper.

To begin healing this language of "not enough / too much," we must begin to heal the wounds caused by the gatekeepers of our past. This is challenging because many of us have become so accustomed to letting someone else have the keys to our stories, but if we are going to take charge of our narratives, we need to take those keys back from those who stole them from us in the first place.

We become our own gatekeepers when we address our stories honestly and, in doing so, release their hold on us. We name the story of the teacher, the friend, the family member, or the religious leader so that we can develop a different story that we don't feel the need to erase.

This is how we heal our stories and own our truth. We stand firmly at the gate with a war cry for all to hear: *I am not too much. I am more than enough.*

WRITE ON THIS:
Too Much and Not Enough

When you think back on the moments in your life when you felt like you were either too much or not enough, what stories come to mind?

Create two lists, one for "too much" and the other for "not enough." Take some time to write down whatever moments, big or small, that come to mind. Include who the gatekeepers were that rooted this belief in you. After you finish these two lists, imagine yourself standing at the gate of your stories, strong and confident, offering a new validation to yourself: "I am not too much. I am more than enough."

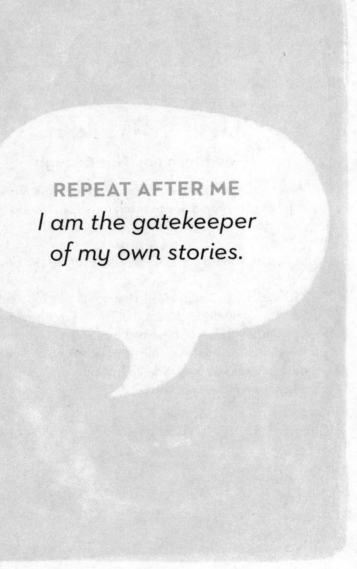

REPEAT AFTER ME

*I am the gatekeeper
of my own stories.*

PART 2
SAFETY

Find Your Edges

When my stories began rising to the surface, I experienced several trauma responses along with them: fight or flight, freeze, and fawn. My flight was sort of an out-of-body experience in which it was difficult for me to stay grounded in my present moment.

"Find your edges," my therapist would say as my body began to fly away whenever the words between us felt impossible to face and triggered something within me that I wasn't ready for. I knew it was happening because my head felt foggy and my body weighted like lead, and yet even with that heaviness I could transport myself mentally while remaining physically in the room.

The first time I was given language for this—*dissociation*—I remember heading straight for the books to search for its etymology, desperate for words to explain what I'd felt most of my life. I read, in bold, "Dissociate (v.). From the Latin *dissociatus*, past participle of *dissociare*, 'to separate or disunite.'"[1] *Separation*, that was it, this feeling my mind was separate from my body; that in a moment, I could be an apparition of myself without any stable container to ground me.

"Find your edges," she said again. "Feel your feet on the floor, look at your hands, count your fingers, blink your eyes, wrap your arms around your shoulders." And so I did, locating all the parts of me and their connections to each other. Little by little, I felt a sense of returning, like a spirit hovering over the hospital bed falling back into its body to revive it. Within these edges, I could sense where I was, a therapist's office with light blue walls. I could tell what year it was by reading the calendar on the side table. I could see my adult hands and know I was no longer a child. If dissociation was separation, finding my edges was integration, my many pieces forming a whole.

Before I knew about dissociation, I judged that splitting within me and felt shame for my memory gaps (sometimes small and sometimes gaping over years), my struggle to stay present during sex even while being in a safe and loving marriage (raising the question within me, Was I a voyeur or a participant?), and my emotional absence when grief was unmanageable (turning on a robotic switch when my emotions were inaccessible). However, finding language for my experience that explained and normalized it removed that shame so I could begin to love and accept myself without judgment.

We all dissociate at various levels, from the mildest versions we experience when daydreaming, scrolling on our phones, or zoning out during a conversation to more involved dissociation such as memory gaps, depersonalization, and derealization (where a person becomes unattached to their own body or their surroundings). The latter form of this intensive dissociation usually stems from early trauma or post-traumatic stress.[2] For those who experience profound dissociation, it can feel as if the edges of their person or environment have gone missing, leaving them vulnerable to falling off into an emotional abyss without a border to hold them. That is why it is so essential to have guardrails to hold on to when we are dealing with stress, recalling past trauma, or navigating hard stories.

I experienced these guardrails in real life during a beautiful summer hike at Glacier National Park in Montana with Landon. We have always loved the outdoors and try to make a trip to explore a new hike each summer. We were on the High Line trail, something on our bucket list we'd wanted to try out.

As we made our way down the trail, it was apparent we were in for a stormy trek on a hike that was already known to be precarious at various points. The rain started out light, then grew heavier as the path narrowed to a steep edge. The rock underfoot became slippery. We held onto the roped guardrail as we continued, and the rain turned to fog so thick that I couldn't see my hand when I held it out in front of me. I gripped the rope harder. The drop-off that had made me dizzy only moments before was now lost in the dense gray. But we made our way along the narrow trail, one small step at a time, holding the guardrail, until the trail expanded and moved us away from the edge—and the fog cleared, revealing an expansive view.

I think about this imagery often when trauma responses rise up during story recovery. There are some parts of the journey that will be steep, even dangerous, where we need a stable rope to hold on to, and other times where the story will take us inland, away from the edges, where we can rest and feel secure. Both are part of the process, and both offer us a view we would have missed if we'd avoided the trail altogether.

When I am helping my clients explore their story healing and writing as a way to process, it is essential to find those guardrails so that they can feel safely contained before the fog settles in. "Feel your edges," I say, as my therapist said to me. "Feel your feet touching the ground, blink your eyes, look at your hands and recall your age, and wrap your arms around your shoulders to feel the borders of your body." It is a straightforward prompt, as it should be. Often, when we are overwhelmed, we have barely any capacity for learning a new breathing technique or meditation; we just need to be reminded that our bodies are in the room and that we are safe there.

In the same way we find our edges within our bodies, we can also find them within our personal stories as we write them down. For example, some folks I work with are writing memoirs and looking for a structure that can serve as a map. They may want a scripted template for their book, but I offer a more flexible, simple framework: Act 1, Act 2, and Act 3. This provides a lot of room for spontaneity within the structure. I am not a fan of tight, immovable outlines, but I am in support of flexible ones that offer bendable borders. To have rigid edges in our storytelling could cause a sort of claustrophobia that can shut us down. Just as our bodies are soft and pliable, so should our creative writing be.

By finding our edges in our storytelling, we can also find more clarity, containment, and freedom in our making. Without these edges, we can fall into that same sense of dissociative separation at the sheer overwhelm of exploring our stories. We can experience cognitive overload (a.k.a. analysis paralysis), which comes when we have so many ideas and thoughts thrown at us that we just shut down altogether like a computer whose drive is packed full and burning hot. How do we fix it? We clear space, delete files, and shut the computer down so it has a chance to restart.

When that overwhelm comes through in writing our stories, it's an important reminder that we need our edges in place—both through an embodied practice and a writing framework that allows us to feel that safe sense of containment. To this day, I keep the words "find your edges" and a sticker of the simple framework of Act 1, Act 2, and Act 3 taped on my desk as a reminder that just as a frame holds art in place, so containment holds our stories as we navigate them.

As I studied the impact of writing down our stories and considered the edges we need to feel safe as we explore our narratives, I came across the work of social psychologist James W. Pennebaker, who became curious about the effects of repression and holding secrets and researched what happens when people begin to write through their emotions. In *Opening Up by Writing It Down*, he says, "Disclosing or confronting a trauma helps us understand and ultimately assimilate the event. By talking or writing about a secret experience, we are translating the event into language. Once it is language-based, we can better understand the experience and ultimately put it behind us."[3] In his research, he found that after participants in his study wrote candidly about painful events in their lives and how they felt about them, they experienced physical and emotional release. This resonated deeply with me. I'd always found writing to be a safe outlet, journaling to see how I was feeling and releasing what was being held in. I knew how it could act as a safe and secure container, offering edges to reflection so that the deep water wouldn't feel like a torrent.

Whenever I and other writers I support need edges and guardrails in our story healing, I consider this practice of expressive writing as a useful tool. We begin with a writing prompt, a specific amount of time (ten, fifteen, or twenty minutes works well), and a journal to freewrite about the prompt. After we have finished, I invite us to a simplistic and symbolic act of containment—we close our open journals to see the words we've written are held between the covers. Our stories are not loose and without edges; our words are contained. We are contained. We are both safe in our telling.

On the other side of the fight or flight response to trauma is the freeze response. Just like the dissociation of flight was something I knew well, so was the freeze. Like an animal that plays dead in order to survive or becomes paralyzed as the headlights face it head-on on a dark highway, it is instinctual for our minds and bodies to enter fear paralysis until they know we are safely out of harm's way. Some experiences take us years, decades, or even a lifetime to thaw from.

Does a similar freeze take place in our story healing as we navigate past pain and try to write the unsayable stories of our past? Yes. So much of approaching the truth of stories exists in facing off with our fears and confronting important questions, such as, Is this safe? Can I put myself out there in the world? Will it be too much for me or for others?

In the same way we need safety and containment to heal past trauma, we also need safety and containment to heal our stories as we write through past pain. During my initial story healing in processing my trauma, my mind felt overwhelmed and my body mimicked the freeze response I'd experienced at the time of sexual assault, paralyzing me. I could not make any movement in writing my stories until I found my edges within my writing practice. These edges were about creating a safe, embodied space for my stories so that I wouldn't retrigger myself in the process.

Setting up these edges looked like having a sacred writing space with privacy and a limited amount of clutter to help me avoid feeling overwhelmed, creating a ritual before and after my writing that included lighting a candle at the start and blowing it out at the end to mark a clear beginning and end of a session, blessing my body and the page with permission to step away if my feelings became too pronounced, thanking myself after writing with a hug to ignite compassion and care for whatever I was about to do that day, and lastly, bringing myself back to the present whenever I felt myself being triggered by the material by drinking sips of water, breathing in and out, standing up and stretching, and humming to create a soothing vibration in my body.

This practice of finding my edges wasn't learned in a single writing session. For years, I felt like I needed to push through and write the hard things, even at the cost of my own retraumatization. Over time, however, as I allowed myself to slow the process and take care of myself, this writing became a way to hold myself the same way a safe therapist or friend would. It's essential to remember that we are writing to create safety and containment for the body's stories.

In a world full of screens and dissociative markers, it is so easy to lose ourselves—whether that is from casual dislocation from scrolling social media or from a trauma that caused us to split off from our bodily experience. When we practice writing, we are invited to return home to ourselves. This is an embodied experience of feeling the texture of the pen, the paper, the hands on the keyboard, the tinge of discomfort in the wrist from writing so long. Putting pen to page is always an embodied practice. Overall, writing can be a practice of trauma-informed care as we begin listening and engaging with the here-and-now experience of the body's story. And is there a more powerful way to heal the wounds of our lives than by tending to them?

When I began sharing the practice of finding our edges with my clients, do you know what finally happened for them? They showed up to their stories with kindness rather than a forced timeline and curiosity rather than contempt. There was a thawing effect on the frozen stories within them. I cannot reiterate this enough: when you're writing personal stories, you are an advocate for your lived experience. And what is an *advocate*? One who supports, defends, and protects an important cause. By showing up to the page to listen and reflect on your life, you are offering yourself the safety and protection you need and have always needed.

Beyond fight or flight and freeze, there is also what's known as the fourth F in reacting to trauma: the fawn response. Psychotherapist Pete Walker, who coined the term, writes that "those who fawn tend to put the needs and wants of others ahead of themselves at the cost of the health, protection, and compassion for themselves."[4] This fawn response is an extension of the freeze response, but instead of a physical reaction, fawning is an emotional reaction to the fear of conflict, neglect, anger, or abuse.

Mostly, this response is learned at a young age through taking on the family roles we spoke about earlier, like the golden child, the scapegoat, and the caregiver. These roles teach us to respond in certain ways to specific environments that bring fears to the surface, such as by offering levity to a conversation to avoid a confrontation, people-pleasing to avoid rousing anger in another, or suppressing one's emotions to avoid shame, blame, or disappointment.

It took me years to notice that the fawn response was my go-to from an early age, and one I still defaulted to as an adult. It wasn't until I had language for this fawn response, learned in a therapy session, that I could begin generating a compassionate understanding of my experience as someone who could acknowledge the assault, release the self-blame, and thank my body for responding in a way that it needed to in order to survive. Before I gained this knowledge, I had blamed myself, thinking the sexual assault I experienced was my fault or that

I must have in some way asked for it. But when I could zoom out from my experience through gaining perspective of why someone's brain and body would fawn as a form of protection in a harmful situation, I could begin to bless the actions of my body rather than curse them.

Fawning has also shown up in my writing and in the writing of so many I have supported over the years. We would censor our voices, holding back on telling the full truth of the story, dismissing the heaviest of our emotions to make the words more palatable—especially for those whom we were most scared of offending. When I started publishing personal essays, I witnessed myself falling into that familiar role of wanting to make everyone comfortable and at ease with my writing—but the cost was sacrificing the truth of my own experiences, memories, and, most importantly, my voice. The process would go something like this: type something honest / delete / write something approachable / delete—until I looked at the pages of my life and asked myself, *Am I willing to release myself from being the caretaker of others so that I can finally be the caretaker of my own story?* This question has been a tipping point for me and for my clients and continues to be one every time we write about our lives.

"How do I write my stories without hurting those I love?" my clients often ask. I watch their eyes well with tears as they share how many years they have put off writing because of the fear of retaliation. I know this question well. And while it is important to consider, I invite us all to ask ourselves another question: *Who am I still protecting by holding back my voice, and why?*

Recently, this came up with a client whose story brought up a memory involving her parents. I could tell she was holding back. She would write something brutally honest, then slide away from the emotion into logic or subtle self-blame to avoid the hard story she was trying to get across. It was as if she was writing with armor on. I wondered who she was wearing it for—herself or others.

"Who are you protecting?" I asked her, meeting her eyes as if in a dare.

Without hesitation, she replied, "My mother."

This admission broke something within her, a wall of fear that had been unacknowledged in her writing until that moment. By speaking it aloud, she gained a new understanding of who she was covering up for through her words. She could now either begin releasing this attachment to her mother's potential retaliation or write her truth around it. And so I asked her, "What is more important at this point in your life—candidness or censorship?"

She wasn't writing anything malicious, any revenge text or unprocessed rage; she was writing a reflective and powerful personal experience. But because she was still developing trust in her story, that fear of retaliation was also present.

I knew this fear as well. When I began writing about my life, it felt like every word was breaking down a wall within me that had been erected to keep me from dealing honestly with the people in the room I'd tried so hard to ignore. This had profound spiritual meaning for me, as though the Jericho walls guarding my heart were finally crumbling to the ground as I marched around them, declaring my stories. With these walls coming down, it meant exposure, vulnerability, and the trauma of sudden change. Though this breaking was essential for my process, I also had to relearn a sense of safety so I wasn't buried beneath the rubble of retraumatization and had to keep finding my edges to remind myself that I was no longer stuck in the past but was alive, present, and safe in this very moment.

It took me years to recognize the way patterns of trauma response showed up in my story healing and writing process. Understanding the fight or flight, freeze, and fawn responses offers us a greater understanding of our past stories and how to revisit them with a process that includes awareness, permission, and safety. When we can see our writing and storytelling through this trauma-informed lens, then we can liberate and thaw the stories that have been frozen within our bodies over the years, offering them the caregiving they need.

Remember, you get to caretake your stories now and offer them the advocacy they deserve. I've discovered there are simple ways to set up an environment for your story healing that can support any fight or flight, freeze, or fawn responses that may show up. I hope that considering your own stories and the process of writing them down inspires you to create a story survival guide of your own, and I have created a list below to help you begin. Please note that there are entire books written on this that are far more detailed, but I wanted to offer my favorite approachable avenues of trauma-informed story care that are accessible for you today, without having to learn any new somatic meditation or technique.

1. *Engage your senses.* Bring sensory experience into your writing space to make it a safe and beautiful environment on your own terms. This may include writing by hand to engage touch; activating smell with essential oils, candles, or incense; snacking or drinking to engage taste; listening to ambient music for sound; and using imagery (nature or art) to encourage sight. This will help bring your body back to the moment if it begins to drift off.

2. *Orient to your surroundings.* Choose a color and look around to locate ten different objects that have that color. For example, I choose blue and locate the color on a journal, in an art piece, on the doorframe, and so on. This can help activate the cognitive brain for focus and attention.

3. *Focus on your breathing.* This does not need to be complicated; just intentionally breathing in and out for up to ten rounds will help regulate your nervous system.

4. *Get some fresh air.* Sometimes just stepping away and getting outside can be a game changer. Feel the ground beneath your feet, smell the wet grass after a rainfall, and notice the sensation of the temperature. This change of scenery can help shift you out of a mindset that might be going too deep or too fast.

5. *Write with your nondominant hand.* This will feel strange, but it is a powerful way to tap into your subconscious and is a great stretch for the brain. Psychologically, it is a powerful support as well. Art therapist Lucia Capacchione's research shows that writing with your nondominant hand helps with stress and anxiety and is also a great way to access the voice of your inner child.[5]

WRITE ON THIS:
Trauma Response Survival Guide

There are so many ways trauma responses can show up in our lives and in our writing process. These responses are innate and essential to understand as protective mechanisms from past pain. Consider the different responses—fight or flight, freeze, and fawn. Which have shown up in your life, specifically as you write your stories? Perhaps, when the writing gets tough, it triggers a flight response, and you run away from the page in avoidance. Or you are in the midst of creating something brave and your body's stress signals go on alert at the familiar sense of danger, and a flight response causes you to dissociate when writing hard things. Or, when you are starting to write that book you've been dreaming about, fear sets in, and you feel paralyzed in a freeze response and call it writer's block. Or perhaps you want to write about your life but are afraid of retaliation from family, and as a result you write around the truth as a fawn reaction in order to placate your rising fear.

Which trauma response most often arises for you in your writing? Try creating a short, trauma-informed survival guide for yourself to avoid retraumatization and provide self-care. This might look like a simple meditation in which you practice being present with your stories when you feel the flight set in and using grounding body techniques to find your edges when you feel triggered by writing tender material. By having wisdom around your responses and how they affect your story healing, you can approach yourself with compassion and self-care.

REPEAT AFTER ME

*I am finding my edges
and creating safety
as I write my tender stories.*

Creative Consensuality

Not long ago, I was invited to speak at a conference about trauma-informed writing. I looked at the hundreds of faces, people with pen and paper in hand, hungry for an answer that would give them a task list of how to heal through writing and how to do it quickly. I recognized a desperation I had known as well, one that had caused me to sign up for what every catchy headline that promised a remedy to recover my stories offered: "How to Get Unstuck and Unlock Your Creativity," "The Only Meditation for Writer's Block You Will Ever Need," "The Essential Trauma Tools to Help You Heal Your Life." Oh, if only creating a how-to checklist for healing was that easy! Some were a little helpful but mostly offered formulas I'd need to learn and apply when I already had little to no capacity for developing a new technique. How I tried, though! I sat through thirty-minute meditations I was too dissociated for and memorized other meditations that felt way too complicated for my already overloaded mental state.

Ultimately, I'd reached the limits of how much I was able to process in a single moment.

I like to think of our limited cognitive capacity as something comparable to a deflated balloon—once vibrant, light, and eager to float away. Still, even if a passerby or angsty kid hasn't popped it, the balloon will deflate on its own in a few days, sometimes less. Then it lies on the floor lifeless, its saggy body completely done with "being." Do you know the feeling? Like that deflated balloon, when we are drained of energy and emotion, the last thing we can think to do is create a task list for our writing or healing journey. We can't even seem to pick ourselves up off the floor.

Over the years, I've found there are several reasons these limits arise in our story healing. *Why* we arrive there is that we push too hard, past something called our "window of tolerance." *How* it shows up is as burnout, depression, and trauma triggers that cause our nervous systems to feel dysregulated and deflated, just like that saggy balloon.

The window of tolerance concept was created by Dr. Dan Siegel, who posited the ideal zone of a functioning state amid stressful or traumatic situations.[1] What he found in his research was that outside this window of tolerance, there are two states we can slip into—hyperarousal and hypoarousal. Hyperarousal is a state of overwhelm, anxiety, and a sense that we have lost control and need to flee the situation. Hypoarousal is the opposite end of the spectrum, when the body and mind shift into a zoned-out, dissociated state because the stress is too much. Our window of tolerance exists as the middle place, where we can be in a state of balance.

Every person has a default zone based on how they learned to deal with stressful situations during childhood. Some tend toward a hyperaroused state—anxiously aware—while others lean toward being hypoaroused—disconnected from their experience. It's so important for us to know our default zone so we can better care for ourselves as we excavate stories that have shaped us.

I have personally experienced falling out of my window of tolerance so many times that now I can recognize the pattern, what triggered it, and how to pull myself back into better balance. In my writing—while facing something that is painful or that feels like too much—I know when I've shifted into a hypoaroused state because I'll slip into a mental fog, become sleepy, and walk around only partially present to the world.

If I know I'll be diving into painful stories, I can bring in objects that help me stay connected to my body—candles, ice water, snacks, cozy socks. I can drink and nibble to keep my body present, inhale the fragrance of a candle, and rub my feet on the floor to feel what is beneath me. I can take breaks often to clear my mind and make other choices to keep myself in a state of self-care. Maintaining this window view, combined with the similar practice of keeping my edges, allows my process of writing to last longer and be sustainable in the long-term.

There is often a mad rush to the finish line in nearly every area of our lives, including our healing journey and story writing. Our hustle culture says we should do more in less time, including creative output, even if that output touches on emotionally tender material. This is dangerous ground to entertain, because if we're trying to race through our story healing, we can miss out on the cues our bodies give us to slow down and pace ourselves as needed.

Not long ago, I played the same game when I told Landon, "I have a killer deadline coming up." I had said the word *deadline* a million times before, but at that moment the word felt different on my tongue—sour, twisted, and totally inhospitable.

When I looked it up, I was shocked at its origin story. According to Merriam-Webster, its use originated in the early 1860s with the harsh definition of "a line drawn within or around a prison that a prisoner passes at the risk of being shot."[2] Some of the earliest mentions of *deadline* are preserved in diaries kept by captive soldiers during the Civil War. It wasn't until years later that the meaning of the word evolved to apply to work culture as "a date or time before which something must be done," and specifically to the world of print media. After discovering this, I decided I wasn't going to use the word *deadline* anymore. Story healing was already challenging enough; I didn't need morbidity attached to my process as well. Instead, I began exchanging the word *deadline* for *lifeline* because that's what story work is. We reach for our healing with intention, risk, and vulnerability; in return, our stories make us come alive.

The etymology of the word *lifeline*, not surprisingly, has a completely different tone. Its first definition, from the year 1700, is "a line (such as a rope) used for saving or preserving life," which refers to the ropes used to save the lives of sailors on vessels in bad weather.[3] This meaning of *lifeline* has resonated with me even more than I thought it would. So often, I think of writing our stories as going for a deep dive, swimming the currents, and learning to navigate the hard elements. The water and the lifeline take us to our depths and also bring us to the surface when we are submerged for too long.

This is why I am a big advocate for allowing our story healing process to be slow and safe, and for consensuality to take the forefront. By *consensuality*, I mean that we get to decide how we heal our stories and the pace at which we engage them so that there is safety in our process. This is so important, especially for those of us who have been impacted by little and big traumas that have taken away our choice and agency. Whether this nonconsent happened to us once, twice, or was an ongoing experience, we can reclaim our agency in adulthood as we begin setting choice and safety at the forefront of our healing process.

Ask yourself this fundamental question: *What do I have the capacity for today that will allow me to feel energized and embodied tomorrow?* Pin this question somewhere you can see it often to check in with yourself. You don't have to push yourself to heal on anyone's timeline but your own. And you get to decide the means and the methods that work for you.

Overall, I've noticed two primary ways we can engage consensuality in our story healing: through the body and through language.

First, the body gives us nudges about choice when we begin to listen to the cues it offers us as we are on the edge of exploring something tender. These body cues are unique to each person but can look like feeling flooded (like your brain is filling up with water), having difficulty breathing (like your chest cavity is filled with weighted stones), feeling knots in your stomach brought on by anxiety (like a rope gathered and tangled at the base of your belly), and so many more. When these cues show up, we must begin to listen to them if we want to prevent ourselves from leaving our window of tolerance and entering a state of stress response. This can be hard to do when we have practiced the art of ignoring the body's warning signs for years, out of habit.

Every body is different. My body commonly speaks to me through a heaviness in my lungs, making it hard for me to breathe. I can tell I am on the edge of anxiety because my breath becomes faster and my chest begins to tighten. When I feel this happening in the midst of my story healing, I am reminded to create safety for my stories. *Will I pause and care for myself here? Will I check my emotional temperature for what I am available for today? Or will I ignore this body cue and keep going anyway?* When we listen and choose to care for our bodies when they speak, we create a consensual, trusting relationship with our spoken and unspoken stories.

To begin to listen and recognize these cues from the body, we need to reflect on how our bodies have responded when they felt stressed, overwhelmed, dissociated, or out of control. Then, while engaging our stories, we notice when our bodies begin sending us similar notes under the door we can respond to. Notes like, *Do I need to pause here? Am I still present? Am I allowed to take my time?*

This embodied listening reminds me of the important "safety stops" scuba divers use to avoid decompression sickness, commonly referred to as "the bends," which in serious cases can be fatal. When divers ascend too quickly, their bodies experience an abrupt decrease in barometric pressure, causing nitrogen dissolved in the bloodstream to form bubbles that can block blood vessels.[4] Divers avoid the bends by taking safety stops on their way to the surface, pausing for a few minutes every so often to allow the nitrogen to absorb and the body to acclimate.

It came to me, as I was feeling flooded in my own writing and story healing process, that I too needed a slow ascension and safety stops in my process so that my brain and body wouldn't be overwhelmed. These safety stops in my writing are simple, as I mentioned earlier. I pause my writing, take intentional breaths, feel my seat beneath me, and then, when I'm ready, I begin my ascent from the deep back to the surface. I keep this practice of safety stops close to me as I'm writing stories, and I share it with my clients when they come to me feeling flooded through their story recovery.

Second, we can practice consensuality through interpreting the language that shows up in our process—language that often includes words associated with violence. I take note when such words arise from my clients who are writing their tender stories and find themselves in a creative block. They typically say something like this:

"I am totally stuck; I just need to break through."
"I have to force myself to show up to the page if I am going to get anything done."
"I am exhausted, but I can push through to the finish line."

Break. Force. Push. When I hear these words, I am taken back to moments of my own experiences of harm, abuse, and silencing. And if I am taken there, what about my clients, albeit subconsciously?

When these words show up in our story healing, they are offering us an important cue, just like the body does, about what we may need at this time. Instead of breaking through, can we gently knock? Instead of forcing ourselves, can we pause and take a breather? Instead of pushing through a barrier created for our protection, can we wait to see a crack form in the wall that we can enter through?

Learning to listen to our bodies and language cues as indicators of when our trauma response might be firing up gives us an opportunity to offer safety for our stories before we escalate to a full-on trigger state. I've found it is often not the intrusive recollections themselves but rather how we respond to them when they appear that is at the root of becoming triggered. Will we be supportive and affirming when we are invited to slow down instead of angry and annoyed? Befriending our stories through choosing to listen and care is how we create consensual self-care for our healing process.

I reiterated the importance of consensuality during a conference I was teaching at recently about trauma-informed writing. I spoke about the importance of slowing down and the antihustle culture that must exist within our writing. I watched these writers fidget in their seats as I called them to pace themselves instead of speeding through their process. It was apparent that they wanted me to give them the most direct way to heal from trauma through writing with an easy bullet-point list, an affirmation to memorize, or a simple breathing exercise—and how to do those as quickly as possible. They had paid and carved time out from their busy lives for this event, after all, but I had no quick fix for them, no shot of resolution, no 1-2-3 hustle toward the finish line . . . on purpose.

I went on to share with them that writing is not a sprint; it's not even a marathon. *Well then, what is it?* their eyes pleaded, pens ready to record inspired wisdom.

I paused and said, "It's a nature trail!" Smiles spread across their faces as they erupted with laughter. There was a notable shift in their emotions, from angst to relief that they didn't have to hustle through their creative process, healing journey, and story work.

The process of writing our stories, I believe, should be the shining example of antihustle culture. It is not a marathon; it is a nature trail.

A nature trail says to slow down, stop, look at the flowers, and take in the feeling of the elevation, the way the air changes as you climb higher, and the resistance you feel when the incline becomes so fierce that you wonder why you attempted this hike at all. Thinking of writing as a nature trail encourages us to ditch the goal of finishing the run in under an hour and instead practice the gift of just "being" with ourselves in a world that says *create faster*. When we allow ourselves an unhurried pace in our story healing, especially when writing hard things, we can give ourselves a chance to have creative capacity without experiencing burnout, overwhelm, or triggers that shut us down altogether.

This approach may seem frustrating, but it teaches us to create from compassion, empathy, and care so that when our writing gets messy and our wounds start bleeding all over again, we have the capacity and wisdom not to rush through but rather give ourselves the space to recover at the pace we need.

There is a wonderful song by Trevor Hall called "You Can't Rush Your Healing" whose title and lyrics sum this all up so beautifully. I remember lying on the warm floor of a yoga class the first time I heard it. My body and brain were exhausted from my chronic chase to keep up with life. I let the words wash over me as a reminder that I could, if I chose, slow down and let myself feel and heal as I needed to.

The same lyrics return to me whenever I think about my healing and writing process in a culture that says, "Here are five steps to heal your life" or "Write for the masses." Such mantras are inspired by a capitalistic consumer culture that is relentlessly hungry, asking us to feed it even if doing so compromises our creative consensuality. We must remember that story work is cathartic work, and that just as we must not rush our healing, we must not rush writing our tender stories. We need to complete safety stops as we reflect so that we can maintain a healthy balance in body, mind, and spirit as we create.

WRITE ON THIS:

Story Nature Trail

We are all so used to the hustle and bustle of life, but how does that affect our healing journey and story work? Consider what pace might support your process and how you can offer more consensuality to how and what you write so that your story healing can be sustainable long-term.

Draw a sketch of your own story nature trail with milestones (or safety stops) indicating how you can care for yourself as you write and heal your life. For example, my nature trail might have a sign that says "take in the view" as a reminder to reread my words with kindness, another that says "get a pep talk from a dear friend or mentor" as a reminder to share my process with a safe witness, and a third that says "rest stop" as a reminder to take my time as I'm writing hard stories.

Just as I can't rush my healing, I also can't rush my writing and creative process. I am allowed to take my time.

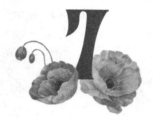

Eyes on the Horizon

My family clambered onto the tiny deck of the deep-sea fishing boat, which did not seem much bigger than a minivan, excited for a full-day fishing adventure in the Atlantic. Such fishing trips were common outings for my brothers when we visited our grandma in North Carolina, but this was the first time I'd decided to jump on board too. The early morning was quiet and still dark, with only the sounds of seagulls squawking as they searched the pier for leftover fish scraps to eat for breakfast. The air smelled of salt water and raw fish, and I felt the waves cause the boat to bob up and down. We untied the mooring lines, took off from the pier, and motored out into the ocean as the sun rose.

We were only thirty minutes out to sea when my stomach began to mimic the way the boat moved, tossed and turned by the ocean. I'd always been prone to motion sickness, but this was next level. It didn't matter how much Dramamine I took, how many copper bracelets I wore, or what number of gingersnaps I nibbled on; the nausea was overpowering.

"Keep your eyes on the horizon," the deck boss said as my little body heaved over the side of the boat. And so I steadied myself, placed my hands on the railing, and looked out past the swelling waves to the sliver of pink morning light where the sky met the water in a seemingly straight line. It was a strange thing to see something so still amid the turbulent motion. He was right; looking at the horizon settled me a bit. Not 100 percent, not by far, but I was able to at least be present for some of the experience.

Years later, I still cling to this phrase, not because of motion sickness caused by boat rides but rather motion sickness caused by life. I pinned this phrase onto my laptop home screen the year I moved to Seattle so that when the waves of a story became so big I feared I might drown, and the rolling emotions came with a cadence that made me feel nauseated, I could look at the words "keep your eyes on the horizon" and be reminded that I needed to be still to heal.

This phrase became a mantra I repeated each week as I took the ferry from Seattle to Bainbridge Island for therapy. I would grab a window seat; that way, I could watch the rain fall as the waves crashed against the side of the boat. I liked seeing the water outside the window, the rocking of the waves against the ferry, the occasional orca whale breaking the surface, and the horizon in the distance. All of it reminded me of the depths I was diving into within my own story healing. I would watch the waves building crest upon crest, the way the white bled into the dark blue seamlessly. I would listen to the crash and roar of the water as it built up and died down with a rhythm that hypnotized me. It was all so similar to what I felt on the inside, like a mirror from the outside world reflecting my inner one—the rising and falling waves of revisiting hard stories.

The ferry ride across the Sound lasted approximately thirty-five minutes, just enough time for me to settle in with my notepad and begin writing. I was working on a memoir about the fractured parts of myself that were being met head-on in therapy. Pieces of me had been split by trauma and made it impossible for me to hold on to a single self. I had parts that felt young and childlike, parts that felt strong and protective, and other parts that felt parental and safe.

I had always felt unable to feel entirely whole. But as I began to write the fractured parts of my stories, it was like inviting all the parts of me to the table. Meeting these parts was akin to connecting with old friends who felt familiar but couldn't entirely be placed—awkward, uncomfortable, and yet often illuminating. This meeting was the epitome of integration work. I took these fractured parts within my writing to therapy sessions, read them aloud, and found that each seemed to hold a specific voice and function. Getting to know these parts was powerful, but it was also painful. With each word came a flood of grief that would rise quickly, making it hard to breathe. There is a common name in therapy for this engulfing wave: *emotional flooding.*[1] It's the idea that you have moved beyond your psychic or emotional capacity in a stressful experience and can feel like you're drowning from the "everything everywhere all at once" happening in your body.

Thankfully, my therapist would help bring me back up to the surface to grab sips of air until the floodwater receded. We did this work repeatedly until my lungs grew stronger and my stamina to handle the flood became consistent. I remembered the phrase kept close to my heart: *Keep your eyes on the horizon.* I have learned to steady myself with a gaze fixed on the line of sky meeting land or sea in front of me or on the line of trees unmoving and still in the distance. I look down at the page containing my words; they sit there confident, bold, and steady, like the horizon, holding me still.

This horizon is much like the edges we seek when we need grounding in our story work. It is connection to our bodies when we feel dissociated, the pause we take when we feel overwhelmed, and the safe writing spaces we create to help us feel contained.

The horizon can be different for each person, but at its core, it is a story anchor in the midst of discovery. To identify your horizon, you must look within and outside of yourself for what helps bring you stability. For me, the horizon in writing is listening to my body's intuition and response. If I notice I start to feel disconnected from the moment, I freewrite by hand about how I'm feeling. If I notice my writing setup is feeling stressful or demanding, I change up my scenery to something that feels energizing, like going to a coffee shop versus an office. Someone else's horizon might look like setting a timer for twenty-minute intervals of writing with breaks to reset or weekly calls with their therapist to talk through what is arising in their story healing. Just as no two people are exactly the same, neither are our horizons.

I keep this practice of looking to the horizon close to me as I'm writing stories, and I share it with my clients when they are in the depths of their own story recovery. I tell them the same thing that was said to me, "Keep your eyes on the horizon," prompting them to steady their minds and bodies on something unmoving so their nervous system can finally catch up with them and they feel grounded again.

"Keep your eyes on the horizon," I whisper, with reminders to breathe deeply and take safety stops often as they ascend from the deep.

"Keep your eyes on the horizon," I say as they write one sentence at a time, allowing time to reveal, feel, and heal as their words invite them to.

"Keep your eyes on the horizon," I tell them as they zoom out from the story they've been sitting so close to that it has become blurry and disorienting.

It is through taking in the horizon while processing our tender stories that the depths we fear can become the depths over which we set our sails in navigating the big waves of our story healing.

WRITE ON THIS:

Eyes on the Horizon

Consider a time you have felt emotionally flooded in your life or writing. How did you allow yourself to fix your eyes on the horizon to create safety and grounding for your process? If this is new territory for you, brainstorm practices that can help steady you in the future. For example: timed writing, sensory support like candles or essential oils, or gentle movement and breathing to reconnect to your body and steady the story waves. These looks to the horizon are how you ground yourself when your stories become choppy.

REPEAT AFTER ME

When I feel the floodwaters rising, I will fix my eyes on the horizon and steady myself.

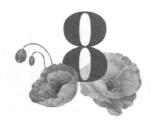

Can I Get a Word Witness?

Growing up in the South, I was surrounded by sermons that echoed from the radio and television. I'd often hear a question that, to this day, sticks with me when I'm writing and helping others uncover their story: "Can I get a witness?" The preacher would shout the question, hands raised wildly, brow sweating with excitement. A witness, a confirmation, a validation, an amen to something being said. It is a question I see repeated subconsciously in the sacred story work I do. And so I became curious: what was the definition of the word *witness*? There are many meanings, but I was struck most by the language of "[to] bear testimony . . . [to] affix one's signature to (a document) to establish its identity . . . to see or know by personal presence, observe."[1] This was exactly what I experienced when I sat with folks writing their stories. They were asking themselves and others, Can you see me? Do you want to? Will you be a witness to my words?

This witnessing through writing and art has existed in me since I was young, though that wasn't the language I would have used for it at the time. Writing was a witnessing of my truth, my longings, and my inner ache to be known well. I hadn't intended it, but from early adolescence, I had been gathering people together to witness each other's stories, a preacher in the pulpit of all things story healing.

The first time I engaged in this "witnessing" was when I created an anthology made up of short stories, poems, and essays inspired by kids I was in middle school with. Stories that told about bullying, intense self-loathing, and even abuse that were only safely told by the written word. These were the days before smartphones and social media that measures one's story by the number of likes and followers. Instead, our words were shared via notes folded origami style and passed to one another between classes. For this book, I gathered the words, typed them on an old typewriter, and stapled them together into a little booklet that I still have today. It sits tattered on my writing desk as a reminder of how this work of story healing all began.

My second witnessing time was during my sophomore year of college when a friend and I created a small group for women we called Safe Haven, which gathered early on Wednesday mornings in a cozy room filled with coffee, blankets, and lots of paper. I had felt the draw to begin this gathering after having conversations, one after another, with girlfriends who were sharing about sexual shame and stories of their past. I thought, *What if we didn't have to feel alone in our struggles? What if we could meet together, write, and share stories about what safety means to us in our bodies as women?* Many in this group struggled to know anything in their bodies but a war. The Safe Haven group continued for years, even after I finished my undergrad and others took on the mantle of leading it. It seemed there was never a shortage of women aching to be in a room where they could open their hearts and share themselves without a filter.

The third time, in my thirties, I envisioned a magazine and storytelling platform where women could speak their truth in poetry, art, and essays. I knew so many who had felt silenced over the years, and I wondered if creating a public space that allowed women to roar could be a chance for voice reclamation where there had been repression. I created the *For Women Who Roar* magazine and invited women from around the world to share their voices. Over the past five years, many women have been published, and thousands more have been transformed by the words these women have bravely shared. There, I've witnessed their brilliance with tears that fall hard on my laptop keys, not only because their writing is incredible but because it is so risky and brave.

There are so many more examples of such sacred spaces, but overall, the people in them all ask the same question: "Can I get a witness?" And without a doubt, they do: a witness in a kind reader and a witness in themselves as they see their lives reflected on the page. When we show up to our stories to bear testimony to our truth or sit across from the story of another with an open heart, we are doing the sacred work of story healing through the art of witnessing.

One of the most transformative places I found story witnessing was in a room I designated as the Womb Room. It was a required part of my master's program to practice the core techniques of story work in assigned groups led by a therapist. I had heard about these groups when I'd first started my degree—how we would practice counseling one another, how it would feel like group therapy in a lot of ways, how we would turn our stories inside out, how there would be nowhere to hide. Those rumors all turned out to be true.

The first time I walked into the Womb Room, I noticed there were no windows, only a hazy, dim lamp that sat in the corner on a tiny side table, with multicolored chairs and pasty gray walls. The room was familiar and warm, reminding me of those humid Louisiana days that rose to 105 degrees and caused us to sweat through every layer we wore. My body sweated here, too, as I walked into this room to join my classmates all staring at one another, our eyes wide and terrified of what we might find out about one another and, in truth, about ourselves.

Our group sat in a small circle, knees nearly touching. I surveyed the faces of those I would be sitting with over the next year: Anna looked back at me, the glare reflecting off her glasses reminding me of my mother. Taryn smiled softly, her face soft and round like my aunt's. Jacob talked with his mouth slightly crooked, making me think of my father. Elijah sat tall and friendly but with a slight air of aggression, reminding me of my brothers. And Tanner, our practicum leader, led the sessions with kind, big hands that made me want to fall into them and never leave, reminding me of every man I'd ever wanted to be close with but was terrified to open my heart to.

It was evident early on in these group sessions that something profoundly disruptive was about to happen in how I understood my life. For months, we would gather in this same room to share stories, tossing them back and forth like a game of hot potato. Some were too hot to hold on to, but even still, we would try. Whenever it was my turn to share in the group, I felt like I was being born for the first time, and everyone sitting there was watching it happen. This felt awkward because I was not being born as an infant, unaware of how messy and obscene my birth was. No, I was a fully grown woman, naked and crying out for the very first time. With every vulnerable story I shared, I felt there was a greater dilation, and I wondered how long my story birth would last—or if I would be a baby breached in the process of uncovering memory and truth.

It was hard to stay present. I felt like I floated out of my body and hovered over the room in a dissociative haze, watching the group watching me. Though I can't recall all the words that were spoken, I can tell you about the feeling—and that is, to be honest, the truest thing of all. When I shared my stories, it felt like I was fading away as the scared eyes of my group watched me slowly disappear in the process. And so I would grip the edges of my chair tightly with every word spoken and witnessed until the end of the session; my body would be entirely drenched with sweat, my face flushed, and my muscles burning from the aerobic work of running in place on the inside.

I want to tell you the process became easier over time, that I could stay in the room and not fall back into the stuck place once again, but that just wouldn't be true. Just like my earliest memory, I'd fall into the narrow crack somewhere between the wall and the side of my brother's bed and cry out. But this time it was different; I had witnesses all around. When I cried out, this group, my therapist, my dear friends at the time, my art, my writing, all of them pulled me out from the stuck place where my story was wedged as it was never meant to be.

Over the next year, we did this work of witnessing one another in the group, taking turns birthing our stories and mid-wifing each other's truth. Did we do it perfectly? No, of course not. We were utterly reckless at times, but when we showed up to the Womb Room each week shaking, we were reborn again and again—messy, crying out, but completely seen by another.

This room was one of the first places I was really asked to stay when the flood of feelings came rushing in as I witnessed others, and they did the same for me. But I have had many other Womb Rooms appear over the years—in relationships, creative processes, spiritual deconstruction, and while writing stories.

These Womb Rooms happen for all of us in the story healing we do for ourselves and for each other. These rooms ask us fundamental questions: Will we stay awake for the hard story? Will we be an understanding witness? Will we let ourselves be submerged in the birthing pool and let our stories be born? So messy and yet so alive.

The word *witness* is one I still use a lot these days with my writing clients and within my own writing. Why? Because at its most basic level, the word means *understanding*, and isn't that what we all ache for at our core?

There is a powerful telling in the Gospels about Jesus the night before his death. He was terrified and longing for his friends to be his witnesses during his most vulnerable hour. We are told that while Jesus was in the garden, awaiting his public death, his body was consumed with stress to such an intense degree that he began sweating drops of blood.[2] This rare condition is called hematidrosis, "in which capillary blood vessels that feed the sweat glands rupture, causing them to exude blood, occurring under conditions of extreme physical or emotional stress."[3] He was in a terrifying mental state and didn't want to be alone, so he invited his friends to be there for his most significant moment of fear and despair, saying to them, "I am so sad that I feel as if I am dying. Stay here and keep awake with me."[4]

I think about how brave Jesus was to say this at such a vulnerable hour. Yet, despite his risk in sharing himself, we're told that these friends could not keep their eyes open or bear the weight of seeing their friend in so much pain. Instead, they fell asleep next to him while he wrestled through his dark night of the soul alone. A witness must be ready to battle for the story and willing to fight alongside, keep watch, stay awake, and pray in the hour of suffering.

As if that risk wasn't enough, later on in the Scriptures we see the resurrected Jesus once again vulnerably asking for a witness when he speaks to his friend Thomas. "Put your finger here; see my hands. Reach out your hand and put it into my side. Stop doubting and believe."[5] Jesus called Thomas to be a witness incarnate, to not only look at his wound but put his hands inside the gaping hole. I love this story because it challenges us to step into wounding, not around it; to write into the depths, not skip along the surface. A witness will be involved in the blood and guts of this story war; a witness must not be squeamish.

This is why I say over and over again that words are witnesses to our lives. They reveal us and, as a result, heal us by allowing us to be known by others and even by ourselves. With every story we uncover, write, and listen to, we are on a passage to spiritual awakening, and no enlightenment has ever come about without some trial or transformation.

Perhaps the most challenging part of being a witness is the surprising element of coming face-to-face with our own neglected story, especially if that story is one we have never before allowed to be born, let alone in front of another. To be a witness for others, we must begin with witnessing *ourselves*, listening to our own stories as we write them down and becoming curious at the story invitations that arise all around us and can make us feel deeply at the drop of a hat.

Whether we stumble into a Womb Room, create one deliberately in a small group setting, or cultivate an intimate Womb Room with a close friend or even our dear notebook—these rooms are for any and all who long to heal their stories. This sacred room can be as simple as a story writing practice at the end of the day with yourself, where you write and then read your words back to yourself aloud with zero judgment, only acceptance. Maybe it looks like asking a close friend if you can share a tender story with them because you need a witness to offer a mirror and kindness. Or perhaps it is starting your own Womb Room gathering with others who long to write and heal their stories one at a time. You get to make your room and find your own way.

So, my questions to you, dear reader, are these: When your stories begin sweating drops of blood and shedding tears, will you stay awake? Will you enter the Womb Room? Will you witness your own sacred stories so that you have the capacity to witness another's?

WRITE ON THIS:

Womb Room

What does it mean to be a story witness, not just for others but for yourself? We all have been in different Womb Rooms to some degree—with a friend, a notebook, a safe community where we shared a truth that was hard to face and were offered a reflection through gentle listening and care. Take a moment to write your own unique story of the Womb Rooms in your life and how they have changed you, or how you would like to create a Womb Room of your very own.

REPEAT AFTER ME

I am a story witness for others and for my own life.

Welcome Home,
Prodigal Writer

We all need witnesses, but often the ones we get are not the ones we'd hoped they'd be. When I was young, the witness I wanted most was my middle brother. I was six years younger than him and hungry for him to pay attention to me. There was a lonely ache in me, a feeling that told me if my brother could see me, it would prove something of value in myself. My journals were filled with tearstained notes about how I wished he were my best friend while he was "too cool for school" at age seventeen. I felt as though I couldn't compete.

Still, I loved him this way, with his wild unpredictability, his sad humor, and his love for me that seemed to mainly show up on late nights when we would go outside and sit on the roof of his car after the rest of the world was asleep. While we'd watch the stars shine late into the night, he would share stories, and

I would listen and ask questions like a little therapist. "How did that make you feel?" "Can you tell me more?" He would tell me many things, and I reveled in his openness with me. To say I looked up to him was an understatement; I thought he was the coolest person in the world.

I wrote my brother several letters around this time, many of which I planned to give him, but they mostly ended up tucked away in the back of my diary for fear of being too vulnerable. These letters were what I longed to say to him, what I wished existed between us, casual make-believe conversations that resembled what I remembered us being like when we were younger. Letters full of mischief, like when we were on family road trips and would press our faces and tongues against the car windows to get responses from passersby; our parents would yell at us to stop, but we'd keep doing it anyway. Letters full of hope, like on Christmas mornings when I'd go wake him up at 2:00 a.m. to see what Santa brought us because I was too excited to stay asleep. Letters that were full of risk, like on fall days when the fallen magnolia leaves covered the yard, and we would stuff trash bags full and try to jump over them, often failing and falling onto the bags so that they spilled wide open, leaving a mess of beautiful debris.

It was my most vulnerable letter yet that made the cut. It must have been at least three pages long; I rewrote it multiple times to make sure it was legible. Within its pages, I spoke to my brother about how much I loved him, and I asked whether we could be friends for real. I folded the letter carefully, and on the outside I wrote in careful cursive, "To my brother, Love, Megan," and slid it carefully under his bedroom door while the lights were on.

Why I decided to do it the day he had a girlfriend in the room is beyond me; it was an inevitable setup for rejection.

I stood outside the door to hear if he saw my gift. After a few minutes, I heard the sound of muffled footsteps and his girlfriend asking, "What's that?"

I could hear the paper unfolding in his hands, one crease at a time. Then there was silence. I waited for what seemed like an eternity.

Then my heart stopped at what I heard next—his laughter. "What's so funny? What is it?"

"It's from my sister," he said, catching his breath. "Listen to this." He made his voice small and mousy in imitation of mine, exaggerating the word *love* with swooning inflection. "I just want you to know how much I love you and want us to be good friends . . ." I could hear his laughter; what at one time could be kind was now so unrecognizable. "Oh, man, she is so dumb."

And with that, I heard a crumpling sound as he formed my letter into a little ball and tossed it into the trashcan with a swoosh. They both laughed, and then the room was silent.

I swear I could hear—and feel—something inside me breaking, over and over again.

I ran back to my room, tucked my body in the farthest corner of my closet, away from the outside world, and sobbed for a long time. Eventually I heard them leave. Then I snuck into his room and found my letter smashed into a lonely paper ball in his trashcan. It was like a rescue mission for my words. I fished them out and carried them back to my room for safekeeping, tucking them into the back pages of my journal as an article of vulnerability. I couldn't allow myself to throw that letter away like it meant nothing, when, in fact, it meant everything to me.

I want to say that this story doesn't still hurt, but when I think of my greatest heartbreaks, and specifically my creative wounds, this is at the top of the list. A story that returns again and again when I start a new creative project, finish writing another book, or take that first brave step toward publishing my work—putting my thoughts, ideas, and heart out into the world to be seen as they are. Every time I do, I hear the crinkled-up paper hitting the trashcan and feel my deep longing for a brother's approval rise to the surface. I still cover my ears at the laughter that sounds like an alarm of all the cruel methods by which our hearts can be rejected.

Many years later, I went to a weekend retreat called the Story Workshop with the Allender Center. We were asked to write formative narratives that shaped us and read them aloud to a designated small group led by two therapists. I shared this story and watched these strangers' eyes fill with tears. They echoed back their feelings as they heard my experience. "I feel the heartbreak of that little girl." "I want her to know she is loved and accepted." "I am so proud of her for trusting her voice beyond this moment."

I heard those words spoken but also felt them hit my body and echo like the sound my letter made in the trashcan. It felt impossible at that moment to accept their kindness, and instinctively I felt myself sinking into my chair to avoid their potential rejection. One of the therapists in the room must have noticed my hiding that day because he said something I'll never forget: "Our families are in the room with us every time we address unspoken wounds. When we acknowledge them instead of ignoring them, the narrative loses its original hold on us."

It was true. Whenever I experienced or remembered an instance of vulnerable risk, my brother was there with me. Every. Single. Time. He was there at the root of nearly every fear of failure and fear of success that created in me the familiar sabotage cycle of wrecking the ship before it reached land. Why did I do that? Because the disruption felt familiar—safe, even—while the arrival, the docking, and the attempt at change was—and still is—terrifying to me.

Most self-sabotage begins with a young story that was never addressed. We spend years replaying the same scene, hoping it turns out differently this time. So much of what I've uncovered in breaking through my recycled sabotage stories has been about changing the meaning of this story, letting little Megan grieve that vulnerable heartbreak, and telling her that not every witness for her words will be a hurtful one. Some witnesses will feel like salvation and offer a chance to begin again, while others who are unsafe for our words will feel like death.

Not long after this creative wound occurred, I found a kind witness in my middle school English teacher, Mrs. Bell, at just the time I needed her. I was an insecure kid who shared her most honest thoughts through my composition notebook. It went everywhere with me, pages folded and stained with spilled ink. Often, to pass time in class, I'd write until the bell rang, so absorbed in whatever I was journaling that I would usually be the last to leave.

One particular day, the clock ticked loudly in the corner while classmates passed notes to each other when Mrs. Bell turned her back to write definitions on the chalkboard we couldn't care less about. Every once in a while, she would call on me to answer a question I didn't know the answer to, and my face would turn hot and as red as a tomato. Then I'd lay my head back down on my arm to hide from Mrs. Bell's gaze and decide to, once again, escape into my journal, writing another poem about middle school shame, a very particular hell that churches somehow seemed not to mention.

I must have left her class more quickly than usual that day, because I left my precious notebook on my desk for any and all to read. I spent the next few hours in a manic panic as

I searched around the school, wondering where my poetry could be. Finally, after school, I retraced my steps back to my English class, the one place I hadn't looked, and saw Mrs. Bell sitting at her desk. I knocked quietly on the open door, and she looked up at me with a warm smile, her small-framed glasses tipping down on her nose.

"Megan! I'm glad you came by," she said as she reached into her desk drawer and pulled out my beloved notebook. It was still in one piece. "Is this yours?" I stared at it intensely, wanting to grab it from her and run away as fast as I could, but she held it close to her chest.

"Yeah, I must have forgotten it. Thank you."

She flipped through the pages like she was already familiar with them. "I looked through this journal to find out whose it was and read some of the writing in here. You are a beautiful writer." She stood and walked toward me and pulled her glasses off to look me in the eye. This was the first time I'd seen her without glasses, and I noticed she was pretty, with smile wrinkles around her eyes.

"Oh, thanks," I mumbled, face flushing. I was a mix of emotions: excited, thankful someone liked my writing, and frustrated that she'd read beyond my name on the inside cover and the first page, where I'd written in big, bold letters: "Do not trespass or you will be prosecuted." I'd hoped that threat would deter any who dared to open my journal.

"The thing is," she went on, "I noticed some poems in there that felt pretty dark and made me concerned."

I felt shocked—shocked from being read, being seen, being recognized. I'm not sure if my mouth dropped when she asked this question, but almost reflexively, I smiled back promptly and replied, "Oh no, I am totally fine. I just like to write lots of weird things." My mouth spread into a smile so wide it cramped a little.

Her eyes squinted slightly in skepticism, then she replied, "Oh, okay. Well, if you ever need anything or need to talk about what you're writing, I'm here for you." She placed her hand on my shoulder and gave me a caring squeeze as she handed over my beloved notebook. I clutched it to my chest and walked away, then slipped the notebook into my backpack, careful not to displace it again.

This memory marks one of the first moments I felt genuinely witnessed by someone. Many had read my writing before—friends, parents, cousins—but no one ever saw beyond the raw talent of a kid to the deeper question of "I am hurting; can you tell?" Mrs. Bell saw me that day, read me, and witnessed me in all my layers. She saw through my plastered-on smile, straight through to the heart of a hurting kid who felt invisible.

I will never forget her bravery in asking me that deeper question filled with care—"Are you okay?" I can imagine it took courage for her to take the risk, ask the hard thing, and look deep into the eyes of a twelve-year-old girl who wasn't used to being seen beyond her superficial layers. To this day, this experience reminds me why writing down our stories and reading others' is transformational. With every word, we are allowing ourselves to be seen and be a sacred witness to another.

Both these moments, the hurtful and the healing, are significant teachers in my story healing, even though it has taken many years for me to see it. I am grateful for the lessons they have taught me over time. Lessons like how to resist the easier choice to ignore moments of past pain, especially when they may not seem as significant as others. Or how we cannot begin the work of creative repair, so that we can move forward, if we don't first acknowledge the creative ruptures that shaped us.

The invitation to revisit our old stories can help us evolve into a new kind of witness for our own experiences, a witness who is compassionate, kind, and the safe keeper of letters written and folded carefully and slipped under the bedroom door. A witness who opens the door and lets the writer in to be read and cared for in their bravery.

Above and beyond all of these witnesses, for me the most profound experience of being witnessed has been through the act of writing down my stories. Writing to understand how I feel and who I am in the uncensored, unfiltered body of a notebook.

I still have all of my notebooks in a large wicker chest, pages upon pages of journal entries dating all the way back to 1995. Each one is completely different; each holds a unique story; each describes a different coming-of-age experience in my life. The pink diary with a fairy on the front has a broken lock from the time I lost the key and had to break and enter to get to my own words. The dark blue velvet journal is soft to the touch and has recycled paper made to look dated on the inside. It was the first thing I bought for myself with the twenty dollars I'd saved up in my pink ceramic piggy bank. The multitude of black-and-white composition notebooks are littered with poetry and Lynda Barry–style sketches from middle school about sad things I could only write and draw in metaphor, never speak aloud. The large red spiral notebook has tear-smeared ink from a broken heart and pages filled with fonts that altered erratically depending on my mood. The journal with moons on the cover was purchased at a store in Santa Fe where I fell in love with the desert. The rugged handmade journal has traveled with me across continents and on train trips, documenting many adventures. The leather-bound notebook, a gift from my dad, contains his handwritten encouragement: "Write everything! What you do, what you think, what you feel. You may read it later and be amazed by who you were." Twenty years later, he was right. I am amazed. I am in awe.

What I love about using a notebook as a witness is that there are no others waiting to read it and offer their opinion, no edit or delete button, and no eyes scanning for words to call out or use to accuse. The notebook listens and witnesses us as we are. It captures the interior of a mind before it is told how to be or how to behave.

The notebooks that fill my wicker chest are honest and, for the most part, horribly written, but perfection was never the point. If my house were burning, I would carry all this writing out with me like a life depended on it, because it does. All my ages are wrapped in the skin of language. Yes, our stories are alive; they are breathing—even pulsating. Put your ear deep against the chest of your truth, and you'll hear the heartbeat of your life. We are each a book without a last chapter, a painting that continues to evolve. And, as Madeleine L'Engle wrote so well, "I am still every age that I have been. Because I was once a child, I am always a child. Because I was once a searching adolescent, given to moods and ecstasies, these are still part of me, and always will be."[1]

I've recently returned to my notebook after a yearlong hiatus, and I'm surprised by how familiar it feels. The way my pen slurs across the page is a stroke of memory. Even when I have months and sometimes years of estrangement, those notebooks reflect my life. The point of all my words is purely to answer the evergreen existential question, Who am I? And isn't that what we are all asking and aching to know at our core?

This is why, when people ask me about a cure for loneliness, I'll point to the page. The written word acts as a mirror, reflecting ourselves back to us. We write to discover versions of ourselves, parts of us that were hidden but now can be laid bare on the page. When we see ourselves there, the parts of us that feel alone can speak what had once been silenced.

Every pivotal moment of my writing has followed a breaking point where I can no longer run from myself. Exhausted from the effort, I would return to the page, coming home to myself despite layers of shame that made me run away in the first place. I like to describe the writing process as one of returning. Like a kid who runs away from home, face blotchy, body full of anger, but after a little while, when the internal storm has calmed, comes back ready to start all over again.

It was pretty hard for me to show my emotions as a kid, mostly due to young trauma experiences I didn't have the capacity to express out loud. Instead, when I felt emotions rising to the surface, I would run to the local park and hide in one of the curvy slides people no longer used until my tears ran dry. There was safety and a sense of control in the escape, though it was only temporary.

As an adult, I found myself running away in the writing process as well. It would go something like this: I would start a project full of excitement, my pen moving with the speed of light—until the hard stories sunk in and the page asked me how real I was ready to be. Then I'd take off running once again, not to an abandoned park but rather by hopscotching over to another writing project that felt easier—only to find the same feeling rising there not much later.

And when I wasn't running from writing by jumping to other projects, I was running by resisting, pushing against rather than going with the flow. If you've ever done resistance training, you know how hard this pushing against can be. Every muscle fires up until it burns. When we write from such a place, we might as well be running in place. We aren't getting anywhere. To write well, to write ourselves free, we must name our running stories, what triggers them, and how they manifest so we can practice using our safety stops. We can slow down instead of speeding up and away when the writing gets tough.

One of my favorite running away stories in the Bible is Jesus's parable of the prodigal son.[2] In this story, a young man leaves home, spends all his family's money, and becomes a destitute street beggar. This prodigal is completely consumed by shame but knows if he doesn't return home to ask for help and forgiveness, he might die. On the way back to his father's house, he prepares a big speech filled with curated apologies, but before he can even knock on the front door, his father runs out and embraces him. His father doesn't judge him, shame him, or tell him "Too bad, so sad, you made your choice." Instead, he throws him a big ole party because he is so happy to have his son home again.

I have always related to this story. I guess it's because I've been the "prodigal writer" more times than I can count, abandoning one story after another, leaving them half-finished, and fearful of showing back up again to something that may or may not be received at the end of the day. So much of healing our stories is about embracing the prodigal son within us. We can take the brave risk of returning home after we've abandoned or "failed at" the story or project; we can be the kind father, welcoming ourselves back. We can cry, kiss, and embrace ourselves without question—we can throw a big party every time we show up to the page because we took the risk to return. Then, also like that welcoming father, our words can look back at us with soft eyes that say something like, *I'm glad you're here; I've been waiting for you.* No shame or blame—just open hands like a safe father.

When the words in my journals stare back at me, even after awkward lengths of time, I am seen. When the pieces of my memory start showing up like a missing puzzle, I am validated. When the pains and pinpricks of my body start knocking again, I am embodied. This is the power of writing our stories and letting our stories write us. We become the witness we always needed, we become known, and we become who we are meant to be by uncovering stories once buried but now brought back to life.

WRITE ON THIS:

Witness Stories

When you think about the various story witnesses in your life, the good, the bad, and the ugly, which have been more harmful than helpful? I know this is a tender prompt, so be kind in recalling it. Consider how these wounds have impacted you into adulthood and how you have begun healing those witness wounds from the past.

    After you write this harmful witness story, I invite you to write a separate story about what it means to be a helpful witness for your own life. Maybe that witnessing of yourself is through writing, art, or an embodied movement practice. Think of this witness story like a parable of your own leaving and returning. How could you retell your own experience as a prodigal story?

REPEAT AFTER ME

*I am a story advocate
and witness for my life.*

Inner Child Altars

had a speech impediment when I was around seven, mainly due to poor hearing, a struggle I still have today. This impairment became apparent to everyone in my household as I sat inches away from the blaring television while Mom yelled, "Turn it down!" But even with the TV at its highest volume, I could barely hear it, let alone my mom's voice. The result impacted my voice as letters blended together for me, sometimes erasing each other in a messy tangle. My words would rush from my mouth like a traffic jam, one piling on top of the other until nothing could make it out. I was sent to a speech therapist whose main lesson, especially at first, was teaching me to slow down. Following the speech therapist's guidance, I would try to pace my words, letting them out one by one. Over time, my words began to have breathing room.

But as I sat in therapy decades later, deep in conversations that brought up memories of past trauma, that stutter came right back, like a fire alarm in my body signaling that something was burning and needed to be put out. It only happened when I talked about my past pain, specifically the past I hadn't yet reconciled. With every stutter, I knew I was onto something important, something that would help me arrive at a breakthrough.

The stuttering became so bad it even began showing up in my dreams. One dream, in particular, reoccurred night after night. This dream took place inside my childhood home. On the outside, the house looked small, like a dollhouse, its baby blue paint complete with white shutters. Inside, the warm smell of coffee filled the air, and in the hall family portraits hung slightly crooked and grinning. I wondered if their mouths would begin to move and tell stories they'd vowed never to talk about if I stared at them long enough.

Below the first floor of the dollhouse was a basement that extended into a never-ending corridor with a number of tall doors that had tiny windows. It looked like something straight out of *One Flew Over the Cuckoo's Nest*, where Jack Nicholson's character roamed the skinny psychiatric halls, quickly ducking out of view of the terrifying Nurse Ratched and her colorful plate of pills. Walking down this long hall, I looked inside the little window on the first door. I could see bodies lying on beds completely covered in white sheets, and I felt an instinctual desperation to save whoever was underneath them.

I kicked in that door with a fury, causing splinters of wood and pieces of the metal lock to fly everywhere because, in this dream, somehow I had the strength of a superhero. The bodies on the beds were so still I couldn't even see them breathing. One by one, I pulled the sheets back like I was performing a magic trick. They were all wounded children, from infants to young adults, eyes wide and mouths open as if they were screaming, but no sound escaped their lips.

Then, as I stood over their still bodies, I recognized them as various ages of myself. I tried to speak to them, but my words stuttered. In this dream—or should I say nightmare— the look on their faces haunted me as they watched my mouth, desperate for any words I could say that would hold them. I was powerless to say anything beyond, "I'm s . . . s . . . sorry."

Around the same time that I was having this recurring dream, I was taking a class that focused on the psychology of dreaming and came across the work of Frederick Perls, the creator of Gestalt therapy.[1] Perls had a theory that dreams represented all the parts of the self—the whole, the rejected, and the disowned. To get to know these parts, the idea was to consider every object and character in the dream as a part of the whole person, and I mean everything.

With this theory in mind, I began breaking down my dream bit by bit in terms of the dream elements and what they could represent.

The Dream	The Representation
The dollhouse	A picture-perfect exterior, a mask of what I hoped people would see on the outside in order to distract them from the darkness I felt was behind the closed doors.
The basement	What exists beyond the external and where I dared to face the internal shadows I'd hidden from others.
The long hallway	The long and often arduous journey of healing I was embarking on and the willingness to step into the dark.

The Dream	The Representation
The locked doors	The hard stories I had locked away in my subconscious memory because they felt too impossible to hold in the present moment.
The blankets on the beds	The things that blanketed my past, such as addiction, religiosity, avoidance, and so on, so I could hide from my own hard truth.
The wounded children	Past harms like loss, abuse, depression, and rejection throughout the various ages of my life that I was holding onto rather than healing from.
The person searching	My role as the advocate for my own story who chose to look beyond what others saw on the outside and instead move toward the hurting that exists in places people often forget to look.

When I considered all the pieces and parts, it was clear what this recurring dream was about, who the children were, and what my stuttering was revealing all along. In the dream, I was the advocate breaking down the doors, pulling the sheets off, and discovering the wounded, hidden children where no one could find them. I was also the one being found; I was all of the broken, bleeding, and silenced children waiting for someone to see them, rescue them, and give them back their voices.

This is what I've come to know about the journey of trauma and wholeness: our mind fractures from past pain so we can contain it and keep it from overwhelming us. Like in my dream, we place fragmented stories behind doors until we are ready to face them again. Do you have a story, a dream, or a theme that keeps showing up in your life? Know this: whatever it is that keeps recurring is a knock on the door of your healing. Our work as story advocates is opening that door and leading each of these wounded children within us out of the shadows and into the light.

When I began opening the locked doors in my body for the first time, I felt as though I might drown from the flood of intrusive memories. Do you know the feeling? The waves wash over relentlessly before you can catch even a gulp of air. When the emotional torrent came for me, I thought of the early swimming lessons I'd had as a child, when I would splash wildly in the pool, my little head bobbing above the surface as I tried to tread.

"Don't fight against the water; it will only exhaust you. Instead, relax your body and float; let the water carry you when you start to feel tired," the swimming instructors would say when my breath became short. When I did what they said and let my body stop fighting, I found it could be held by the water after all. I could trust it and let go.

In the same way, when I began to face memories so fierce they made me stutter, I had to allow myself to stop flailing against them and face them one by one so that they could lift me to the surface and liberate me.

It's funny. Those swim lessons of long ago are similar to those I offer my writing clients today when they find themselves pulled underneath the current by telling a hard story. I say, "Don't fight against the story; it will only exhaust you. Instead, stay curious and compassionate. Let your story relax, and it will write you when you start to feel tired."

I've applied these lessons to myself whenever my old wounds rose to the surface, and I've come to the conclusion that if these foundational wounds are rooted in childhood, then so, too, is the foundational healing. I've heard folks talk about inner child healing for years, offering advice like "Connect to your inner child," "Write affirmations to them," or "Love them," but it sounded so ethereal, metaphorical even. This hasn't been the case for me. My dealings with the younger versions of me have always felt alive and completely tangible.

Years ago, I had recently moved, and I came across the wicker chest filled with my journals. I decided to revisit the words of my youth, and I felt a sense of nostalgia remembering who I was when I was younger as I pored over the old entries.

I was rummaging through an old middle school journal written in pencil when I came across a story I had completely forgotten about. In messy handwriting was an entry about feeling overwhelmingly sad and alone. My friends were all mad at me, and deep within my chest was a pervasive dread that felt like it was going to swallow me whole. I described this in detail, sitting in my family's den, looking out the sliding glass doors, tears streaming down my face as I prayed in a fit of despair, "God, please help me. Show me a way out. Give me some light, please. It's so dark here." At that moment, I was a desperate kid afraid of the cloud of sadness that overtook my thoughts.

As I read this journal entry from my younger self and saw the handwritten words blurry from that day of crying, it was a strange thing not to remember this particular day at all. Even still, I couldn't help but feel a deep sympathy for this little girl.

I turned to the next page. It was a drawing, and this time I had a flash of memory as I looked at it. I remembered how, in that young moment of desperation and fear, I'd looked out through the screen doors to see a figure of a woman covered in light, glowing and smiling. She looked just like an angel, the kind my grandma shared stories about. I watched her in awe that day and drew a picture in my journal so that I wouldn't forget her, along with the words she offered that gave me hope when I struggled to find any: "Don't give up, Megan. You have so much life to live and so much to live for. Keep going. You're going to be okay. I am here with you."

As I sat with this journal entry decades later, recalling a moment that had completely been subdued in my memory, I felt the tears fall, just like they had back then. I stared at my sketch of this angel as she stared back at me, with eyes as familiar as my own. Suddenly it was apparent. How did I not see this before? This wasn't an angel. This was an older version of me. I just hadn't recognized myself at the time in the angelic figure I saw before me, filled with hope and a future. I took this journal to the bathroom mirror while holding up the young portrait I'd drawn. She *was* me. She had my face, my eyes, my lips, all much older now, knowing what little me couldn't have at the time—that I would be okay after all, that all the ages of me were supporting my life to come.

So when I talk about inner child healing, it is not a metaphor, at least not for me. When we listen to what our younger selves have to say and hold space for them to heal, we can heal the past, the present, and the future.

Later on, as I ventured deeply into my story healing, I had an idea to connect with my younger self by creating an Inner Child Altar. The word *altar* comes from the Latin *altare*, meaning to raise up, to worship.[2] I wanted to create an altar for my younger self—not to worship myself but honor, bless, and pray for the ages of me that hold stories I can never fully know. After all, she deserves to be honored. She deserves to be raised up.

I gathered dozens of childhood pictures of myself, ranging from a bloody birth photo taken directly after I left the womb to two-year-old me in diapers riding on the back of a pony, to eight-year-old me with a bowl cut and softball attire, to thirteen-year-old me with braces staring snarky eyed at the camera, all the way up to my cheesy senior photo in a green polo shirt leaning against a staged fence.

Photo by photo, I taped them to my wall in order, birth to age eighteen. Below the photos, I set up candles, stacked old journals filled with my early poetry and diary entries, and even displayed some art I'd created when I was little. When I sat before this altar and lit candles for every age, I'd ask the images, one by one, to tell me a story. And they did, often in shy, hushed tones, but if I listened long and hard enough, I could hear them clear as day.

Sometimes, I would take the process even further and read a journal entry aloud, then write back to the child who wrote it like a counselor they could have used at the time. It felt like I was calling back the missing child within me. To say this process of calling my ages together to witness them was powerful would be an understatement. I felt like I was on holy ground.

This inner child work felt sacred; I wanted to create a blessing for my experience. Growing up, in my family we said a blessing for every meal, for trips we would take, and for those suffering or sick. The blessings were a symbol for hope more than anything. In his book *To Bless the Space Between Us*, John O'Donohue writes,

> A blessing is a circle of light drawn around a person to protect, heal, and strengthen. Life is a constant flow of emergence. The beauty of blessing is its belief that it can affect what unfolds. . . .

Regardless of how we configure the eternal, the human heart continues to dream of a state of wholeness, a place where everything comes together, where loss will be made good, where blindness will transform into vision, where damage will be made whole. . . . To invoke a blessing is to call some of that wholeness upon a person now.[3]

The way we engage our past pain, our suppressed stories, and our younger selves is with the choice to bless or curse. Just as we can bless one another, we can also curse one another—one word that means to offer encouragement and another that means to invoke harm. When we show up to our younger selves with compassion and curiosity, we bless the ages within us who didn't feel safe. On the other hand, if we show up to our younger selves with judgment, criticism, and blame, we curse their experience.

When I created my Inner Child Altar and thought of all the words I'd said to myself over the years—mostly mean, if I'm being completely honest—I knew there was some serious healing that needed to happen. I felt that offering blessings for all the ages of me lined up across my altar could aid in this healing, so I decided to write an inner child blessing as I looked at photos of little me. I touched the images of their faces, studying their tender expressions, and felt them reaching right back to me in return as I read these words aloud.

My Inner Child Blessing

I bless you, little one.
The bloodiness of your birth. The first cry.
The beginnings of hunger and longing.
May you know fullness and contentment with your
    desire.
I bless the little fingers and toes.

That reached for a mother, a father, a brother, a friend.
May you know today that you are held by my presence
and care.

I bless the playful innocence of your young soul.
That chased the sunlight before you knew to fear the
dark.
May you know that risk to play once again and heal
through curiosity.

I bless your young body, your skin, your eyes, your
hair.
That began too early to take on insecurity that was
never yours to hold.
May you know your beauty is breathtaking and that
you are loved.
I bless all the feelings that you ever felt or were afraid
to feel.
The feelings of sadness, fear, doubt, anger, love, desire,
and hope.
May you know that all of you is welcome here now.

I bless your voice, from the first cry of birth to your
final growth spurt.
That voice that was silenced, ignored, and told to be
quiet and listen up.
May you know now your voice matters, your stories
matter, you belong here.
I bless your adolescence, your changing body, your
newfound longing.
The friends you made, the friends you lost, and all the
times you felt alone.
May you know you are good and worthy and more
than enough.
I bless all the ages of you and all the ages you will ever
be. Amen.

This blessing is one I return to whenever I feel the waves of emotion crash in, or my stutter returns when I am pronouncing a hard truth. They are the tide of words that come in when I feel that familiar sinking dread I wrote about in my journal, when I needed the voice of an advocate who could remind me of who I was. Whatever your relationship is with the words *blessing* and *curse*, I'd invite you to consider how you can approach them with fresh eyes. How can you begin encouraging the stories within you that have felt shameful and hidden in the darkness? How can you liberate them with a blessing that invites all the ages of you to be seen and known now?

WRITE ON THIS:

Inner Child Blessing

This creation of an Inner Child Altar and blessing have been foundational in my story healing and with many others I've had the privilege of supporting. I invite you to set aside a couple hours to create an Inner Child Altar of your own and write a blessing for your younger self. Think of this as a retreat with your younger selves: getting to know them, listening to them, and loving them. Then, when you finish, read that blessing aloud over your altar to heal the young, wounded stories within you.

Here is a step-by-step guide to help you get started:

Step 1. Make sure this altar has a special space of its own. Maybe it's in a corner of the room, on a desk dedicated to it, or in a closet. The point is that this is a stand-alone shrine for little you.

Step 2. Gather photos from your childhood from birth to age eighteen. If you have a ton of photographs to choose from, select the ones that most speak to you from each age. If you are struggling to find photos at all, use what you do have; even one will work.

Step 3. Gather some things you loved as a child, such as art, dolls, LEGOs, rocks . . . whatever it was that brought you joy when you were young, add that to this space.

Step 4. If you have journals or artwork from when you were young, add this to the altar as well. You will use these materials later.

Step 5. Assemble your altar: put up the pictures, set up candles, and display your young art or journals and the little things you loved. You may also use essential oils or sage to bless the space, if that is part of your practice. You will also want to include a journal and pen to write with as you reflect.

Step 6. Begin to write letters and poems to the different ages of yourself in the pictures, or maybe even write responses to your younger journal entries like you are their friend or caregiver. What did they need to hear that you can offer them now? Read these aloud to each picture. This is your advocacy, your witnessing, your healing. Also feel free to play with the toys and materials your younger self loved, then write about what the experience brings up for you. There is a lot of freedom here. Choose what feels most aligned and sacred in engaging with your Inner Child Altar.

Step 7. After you have written letters to your younger selves, listen for their responses back to you and write them down. This is a powerful exercise because it opens the door for conversation between you and your younger selves.

Step 8. When you are ready, try writing your own inner child blessing. Here are some basics to consider:
• Start with the word "May" for each stanza.

- Write short sentences with lots of imagery.
- Write each sentence on a separate line.

Your blessing can be super short or pages long. It is totally up to you. Feel free to read it aloud over your Inner Child Altar when you're finished.

After this powerful exercise, be sure to rest and take care of yourself. This is a deep dive. Be kind and let yourself restore.

*My younger selves are here
to help me heal my voice.*

PART 3
RESILIENCE

Passing Through Grief Portals

When I was growing up, we visited my grandparents on the inner banks of North Carolina nearly every summer. We spent most days at the Oceanana Pier on Atlantic Beach, which stretched about a thousand feet into the ocean. My brothers and I would walk the long, splintery pier with our rented fishing poles and a box of fresh worms from the market, and either Grandpa Keith or Daddy would help me throw my line in as I watched the waves hit the pier with a force so strong it felt like the whole thing might topple over.

I loved these fishing days but rarely caught anything worth taking home for a fish fry. If I caught anything it was usually a baby shark the size of my little arm or the occasional stingray. I would feel sad for my new little friends, so we'd unhook them as gently as possible and throw them back in the water, and I'd watch the big waves carry them away.

One summer day, however, everything safe about Atlantic Beach seemed to turn sideways. This time, I was no longer on the fishing side of the pier but on the other side, with the strong waves and baby sharks.

My parents went to the store while one of my brothers, Grandma, and I stuck to the beach beside the Oceanana. The sun was bright, and the beach was alive with children building sandcastles on the shore, people fishing from the pier, and the occasional surfer catching a wave. I watched it all, taking in the salty air and the cawing of seagulls as they sailed in the breeze. The current was strong, and the roar of the water seemed to call me into its dark depths.

I had learned to doggy paddle at the local pool just a few months before, and I decided to show off my new moves in my purple polka dot swimsuit that made me feel just like a mermaid. I held my nose and dunked under a big wave to grab a fistful of sand in search of treasure. There was little to hold on to, just broken seashells that slid right through my fingers. The water was a murky turquoise, but I still could see silvery schools of forage fish swim by, tickling my toes, and I chased them, heading farther and farther out. The saltwater burned my eyes. Then I surfaced to find my feet could no longer touch the bottom. I could see my grandma and brother far away, like tiny little dots. As the realization sank in that I was alone, far from any shallow end, I began to beat the water wildly with my six-year-old legs and arms.

My grandma must have seen the top of my head bobbing like a buoy far beyond the sand bar, and she hollered for my brother, who was only a few years older than me, to swim out and get me. I watched him come toward me through my blurry vision, and when he reached me at last, he breathlessly cried, "Get on my back!" I'd done this many times before in swimming pools where I'd begged him to take me on "dolphin rides," wrapping my legs around his skinny waist while he rose up to the surface and then dove deep under the water. But this was different; this wasn't a fun dolphin ride in a swimming pool, this was a fight for our lives in the strong swells of the Atlantic. He began to swim us toward the long fishing pier, but the riptide was especially powerful that day, and he had to fight its pull.

Once we reached the wooden pylons, we both wrapped our young arms around them. It felt like hugging one giant splinter. Holding on, I felt little bites on my toes and wondered if those baby sharks might just come back for an act of fishing revenge. Yet it was the roaring ocean, not the wildlife, that was the greatest threat that day.

Each powerful wave closed us in and slammed us harder into the prickly pylons. We couldn't break away from there. Every time we tried, the riptide would start to pull us back out to sea, so we would grab hold of the pylons again as the only thing that could keep us from being washed away.

On the shore, I could see my grandma on her hands and knees, yelling, "My grandbabies, my grandbabies! Jesus save them!" as she pounded the sand. She was always a praying woman. But swimming? I never saw her swim once that I recall, although I'm sure she would have loved to walk on water that day to save us.

How long were we there? A few minutes, an hour? All I know is it felt like a lifetime. Drawn by my grandma's shouts, a couple of surfers responded and were able to reach us. We climbed up on their boards and lay there, bone-tired, as they swam us to shore.

Scratched up and exhausted, we both fell asleep on the re-clining beach chairs for hours. We woke up to find towels had been lain over us to prevent sunburn and Band-Aids placed on our skin where the wood had cut deep. At one point I heard the soft and distant voices of my parents, who showed up in the aftermath, say something like, "We should have been here."

Many years later, with my heart reconciled and confident in my sense of self, I sat with my momma by the ocean in the Pacific Northwest and watched the waves dash up against the large rocks on Cannon Beach. We talked about that long ago day by the pier, and she shared that my brother had been scared to go in the water with me after that day, and that he would avoid big bodies of water whenever I was near. I didn't blame him.

Even now, decades later, he and I have a vast ocean of things left unsaid between us. I get it. It's hard to go deep with someone you love—into the unknown, the dark roar of emotional depth. To a place you don't know if you will ever return from. That near-drowning didn't scare me, though. Instead, it only made me want to understand the wildness of the waves even more and swim even harder when the tide turns. After all, I've never been someone who was drawn to the shallow end of the pool, literally or otherwise. Instead, I dive headfirst into the depths because I need something of substance, the texture of a truth and not the distant hologram of a lie.

After I had immersed myself in the deep waters of my stories, I was able to see how this near-drowning experience mimicked my own trauma. It is possible to go too far, to get so caught up in the search that you lose the present. I became obsessed with the questions, the nonanswers, the botched memories that slipped so easily through my fingers, making them impossible to hold on to. I went to impossible depths without caution because I wasn't concerned with safety and wasn't even sure it was important, and I suffered immensely because of it. Like the little girl who chased the forager fish as the riptide pulled her out into the ocean, I chased my stories until the waves nearly had me.

You can explore your stories so far into the core of something that it ruptures. You can plunge so deeply into the abyss that you don't have enough oxygen to make it back to the surface. You can do all those things—but you will suffer with your stories instead of accepting their invitation to become alive. I don't want this for you. I want you to heal your stories safely and with edges that sustain you over time.

Please hear me: I want you to swim deep and wide for your stories and truth, but do so with awareness, compassionate care, curiosity, and a steady, supportive pace. Write and create with the care and presence of safe friends to process with, take pauses and seek out the light as much as you seek the dark, and practice being in your body.

You have everything you need within you to listen to your body's story and care for yourself along the way. Story healing, if nothing else, creates resilience, and much of that resilience is developed through learning how to dive into the deep water, rise to the surface often to breathe, and take safety stops to allow your body and mind to catch up with your process. You are allowed to take enough time to swim safely—remember, you are on a nature trail, not sprinting in a race. Your stories are always waiting for you. My story healing process sometimes seems like it has been a series of spiritual awakenings, always at the deep end of something—the end of a relationship (as I knew it), the death of a dream (that had to die to be reborn), the withering of a faith I no longer aligned with (in order to grow again with new roots), the termination of a place (that said it's time to be present in a season of transition).

Theologian Shelly Rambo calls the trauma experience "the 'middle,'"[1] where there is no explanation for the suffering, no positive spin on death, just the silence and stillness of a grave.

This "middle" is not an actual place but a memory from a time that cannot be seen, heard, or touched yet haunts the survivor. There are many other names for this middle space. In psychology, the term used is "liminal space,"[2] the in-between that exists in transitioning from one stage of life to another. The uncertainty accompanying this liminal space is also where we are asked to pay attention and awaken to what is happening within us as we exist there. In writing, this is considered the "messy middle." You are in a writing flow and then arrive at the middle space, and you feel dropped abruptly into unknown territory. This messy middle can feel similar to the strange feelings that arise from not being able to predict the direction or outcome of a story.

In the Christian church is a middle space known as "Holy Saturday." It represents the middle day—the day after Christ's death but the day before his resurrection. This is the darkness and doubt, the giving up, the grief and skepticism of hope. In the most basic way, it is the blank page, the writer's block, and the story's stuckness. The gift of this middle space is the invitation to continue showing up to the blankness and the doubt with an ability to sit with ourselves in silence when no words can suffice.

Whatever name we give to this notion of navigating the unknown—the messy middle, the liminal space, or Holy Saturday—each one serves as a reminder to explore the ocean floors of our own stories with safety so that we can heal moments of grief and loss in our lives.

I think of story healing as the process of traveling through something—a doorway, a bridge, a grief portal to cross to the other side. If you've ever watched *Star Trek* or basically any sci-fi/fantasy film, you can picture these portals: large, circular, and mirrorlike with watery colors that draw you in. These portals show up in places that are often surprising, asking the characters to transport somewhere they might not know or, sometimes, places in the past they recognize. This is why there is so much risk in stepping through the grief portal when it shows up because we have no idea where it might take us. This risk can be utterly terrifying. Before you enter the grief portal of a story, it's critical to check in with your capacity for the emotional risk it may bring. This could be as simple as asking yourself, *How grounded do I feel today? How steady are my emotional waves? Do I have space to care for myself after I dive in?* If the answer to this last question is yes, then swim— and surface often. If the answer is gut-level uncertainty or an outright no, then give yourself permission to return later when you are ready. This, my friend, will expand your capacity to choose, to be safe, and to grow in resilience.

I've gone through many grief portals in my life, but the most profound ones have been through the gift of writing personal stories. It is like writing opens up a passage through denial, through anger, and through depression in order for me to come out on the other side. But just as we must enter the grief portal to heal our stories, we must not remain there, caught in the riptides and nearly drowning from the past.

To recover these ongoing stories, we don't try to change the past. Instead, we sit with the stories and witness them, hold our younger self's hand, and say, "I see you. I am with you now. I am not going anywhere." When we practice this witnessing of our stories, we can find a new meaning for this pain, meaning that exhibits kindness, care, and love for a past heartache we cannot alter but can be present for.

Grief researcher William Worden identified four stages of grief that we all must move through to come out on the other side: acceptance, process, adjustment, and forward movement.[3]

We begin at the road of *acceptance* (stage 1). So often, when grief is new and close by, it can feel impossible to accept. We slip into denial, though not so much as an outright statement like, "No, this did not happen." It is much more subtle than that. Instead, denial can look like avoiding the deeper truth or a vulnerable telling of an experience.

In the *process* of story healing (stage 2), I talk to folks a lot about the importance of writing through rather than around. Writing around something painful is often more approachable because it keeps us safely in the shallow end, but when we write through, with all honesty, we swim into the depths, and that can be terrifying. Author Roxane Gay describes this as writing into the wound. "There is no pleasure to be had in writing about trauma. It requires opening a wound, looking into the bloody gape of it, and cleaning it out, one word at a time. Only then might it be possible for that wound to heal."[4] This is so core to the grief work we must do in our writing; we must address that there is a wound in the first place, then determine how we can begin to provide care for it so it is not left to fester without the attention it needs.

It's hard to go where the truth is, and it can feel much easier to write around it. I want to put flowers around the grave of my buried stories and just observe. I don't want to get into the ground, smell the dirt, and taste its grit. But this is what Jesus did—he went into the dark cave, past the bleeding place, beyond the desperation of hope. He tasted death and died. Then came the miracle, the shaking ground, the absurdity of death, the resurrection. This is what storytelling does—it raises the dead, lifting doubts and beliefs from the grave.

At the heart of it, the process of writing our stories, of grieving, is a series of steps that form a continuous cycle as we deepen our understanding and empathy for the grief in our stories. It is so easy to jump ahead to the ending, to think we're in this for the sake of making a product or reaching a certain outcome, but that is not how it goes. We find one word, then another; we form a sentence, then another, and then another. We learn, we listen, we swim the depths and plunge into the unknown—and we don't forget to breathe deeply.

Recently, I attended a writing retreat in Santa Fe. In the middle of town sat a beautiful old cathedral that drew many inside to pray and meditate. In the courtyard was a prayer labyrinth, a set of circular paths you weave through to reach the center, with intentional stops along the way often used for inner reflection. Walking a labyrinth is prayer or meditation in motion that represents an embodied process of healing and spiritual understanding. Labyrinths have been around for many centuries, and at the core of each is an idea of journeying through rather than around.

Before trying this prayer labyrinth for myself, I did a little research. One labyrinth society, Veriditas, says that there are "three stages of walking a prayer labyrinth: purgation (releasing), illumination (receiving), and union (returning)."[5] These stages resonated deeply with me as I took my shoes off and began tracing the stone path. No one else was around, and it was late enough in the day that the sun was setting behind the mountains in a pink haze. With every step, I breathed, feeling a release of expectation I'd been holding in my body. As I reached the center of the labyrinth, I paused to receive the feelings I had tucked away. The winding process reminded me to take the story cycle step-by-step. Then I slowly made my winding way back out of the labyrinth, a semblance of returning. I did this repeatedly until the courtyard turned dark, and the only sounds were a few people far in the distance.

For years, I held onto my trauma, terrified that if I released my hold on it, then it wouldn't be real anymore. When we choose to explore the depths of our stories, there is a shift that must happen with us, an *adjustment* (stage 3). This transformation can be challenging because we tend to want to hold on to the past pain, thinking that letting go would mean to let go of the experience. I needed my pain to be real because if no one else experienced it, then I was its only witness. Letting go of this belief wasn't an overnight adjustment; it was a long walk back and forth, back and forth, until my feet became weary and said, *Enough; that's enough for now.*

Writer and spiritual teacher Parker J. Palmer writes, "Some journeys are direct, and some are circuitous; some are heroic, and some are fearful and muddled. But every journey, honestly undertaken, stands a chance of taking us toward the place where our deep gladness meets the world's deep need."[6] When we move through this process of grief acceptance, embracing the process, and experiencing the adjustment it creates in us and our world, then we can begin to *move forward* (stage 4), the final phase of grieving. This forward motion is not an ending but a labyrinth of becoming. No longer are we trapped by the past but are bravely journeying through rather than around. We can evolve our stories from the middle place of the scary unknown to a forward place of integration, of understanding where we've been, and of hope for where we are going next.

WRITE ON THIS:

Awakening

When you think about your own journey of story healing, how have you experienced spiritual awakening, such as in the middle space, the ocean depths, the labyrinth, or the grief portal? Try writing your own story of awakening through this process.

Want to take it further? Try to describe or draw a grief portal that you have gone through. What did it look like, feel like, sound like? Feel free to pull out the crayons for this one too. When you finish both of these exercises, take them in. What did you come up with? What are they revealing to you now?

REPEAT AFTER ME

I am created for depth and discovery. My stories are mysteries that I am forever unfolding.

Your Body Is Brilliant

How familiar are you with this popular nursery rhyme? "Humpty-Dumpty sat on a wall. Humpty-Dumpty had a great fall. All the king's horses and all the king's men couldn't put Humpty together again." I remember singing it as we skipped down the sidewalk or bounced to its words sitting on our grandma's knee. We, in elaborate demonstrations, would showcase the "great fall" by jumping high in unison and then collapsing on the count of three, our bodies strewn across the front lawn. Then, stained in green and laughing, we'd jump up and do it again.

One of the other nursery rhymes we loved growing up was "Ring Around the Rosie." "Ring around the Rosie, a pocket full of posies. Ashes! Ashes! We all fall down!" my friends and I would sing as we formed a circle, holding hands and falling down at the end of it with high-pitched squeals of laughter. We didn't know the dark origin of this rhyme, its words illustrating the Great Plague of 1665: the roses the symptomatic rash, the posies the medicinal herbs, and, of course, the ashes the cremated remains of over one hundred thousand bodies that fell from this devastating illness.[1]

Many of the rhymes and fairy tales I grew up with I now recognize as trauma narratives disguised in children's books and songs. "Humpty-Dumpty," in particular, was especially illuminating. You have this adorable anthropomorphic egg sitting high up on a wall, even though he was breakable as hell. Eventually he falls, and his shell breaks into a million different pieces, so much so that no one can put him back together.

We embody this nursery rhyme and many others, these metaphors of trauma, again and again as a demonstration of what happens when we break, a shattering effect sometimes so intense, it's beyond repair.

I remember the feeling well when my own adult body broke apart. I moved into bed at the onset of depression and didn't leave for months, until the seasons changed colors. The room was dark with heavy shades that shut out the Louisiana light. I could hear the coffee brewing and the shuffling of productive feet, but the only energy I could muster was to dig my body further into the familiar cocoon of my comforter.

When I was little, I would sleep beneath piles of blankets, not because I was cold but because their weight felt safe, like soft armor. It was like a game I'd play, lying flat and layering on the blankets one by one, sleeping and sweating, sleeping and sweating. Once, my family panicked because they didn't know where I was—for hours. The phone rang wildly, voices raised in frantic yelling, my mom's feet raced down the hall. Yet, all the while, there I was in my room, covered high with pillows and blankets. Eventually I crawled out of bed and walked out to see my mom's trembling form. "Momma, what's wrong? Who are you looking for?"

We repeat what we know. We repeat what we haven't named. We repeat to protect a story we've been handed. In that bed, as an adult, I was repeating a pattern of hiding I'd learned at a young age. The only difference was that my legs were now too long for this old story; my feet hung out over the metal frame, letting in cool air that hit with a shock. I couldn't hide like I used to—and thank God, because this time my stories were calling me out into the light.

When I finally began to emerge from this warm asylum, my body had *language*. It may seem like this would be a strange thing, but when my body spoke, I knew her voice. It was like talking with an old friend whom you haven't seen in ages, but after an instant of being with them, it's like nothing changed. My body felt like that. It was as though my body was telling me a knock-knock joke—but it wasn't a joke at all.

> "Knock knock."
> "Who's there?"
> "Your body."
> "Your body, who?"
> "Your truth."

My cold feet were only the beginning. I soon felt painful, pin-like pricks and screaming muscles and joints. My head felt like it was in a vice, and my immune system just collapsed. Our bodies speak, and mine was saying *Wake up!* Every week I was in the hospital with some new symptom and zero explanations. As frustrating as it was, this discomfort had me looking at my shattered memory for the first time with a question: *What do you want?*

When we turn to our bodies as storytellers, becoming curious about their torn-out pages, we begin to interpret the truth of our lives. Crawling out of that bed and opening the curtains was the first step for me; the next was paying attention to what was knocking from the inside of me.

The body is brilliant; it took me a long time to know and believe it, but it is a historian, archiving millions of moments, years, and even generations before us whose stories have been passed down epigenetically. It often speaks stories of the past, and in a language we must be willing to learn to interpret.

The first time I was told my body was brilliant was in a dark therapist's office on Bainbridge Island, a room with a maroon carpet and a small sound machine that sat in the corner making bubbling fish-tank noises. My therapist at the time, whom I had been working with for a little less than a year, sat across from me in a tall chair. She had short hair and soft freckles smeared across her fair skin. She leaned toward me, pressing her palms against her long face. "Do you know how brilliant you are?" she asked me, eyes wide and smiling. I felt my body instinctively fold over itself, an intuitive posture I'd learned young and assumed anytime the heat of shame and insecurity arose.

"Do you know how brilliant you are?" she asked again, waiting for my response.

"Oh, was that not rhetorical?"

She adjusted her glasses on her nose and looked at me intensely. "It was not rhetorical. I would genuinely love to know if you can see your brilliance."

I had been opening up to her for months, growing deeper trust in her insight. But with this question, I couldn't shake the feeling she was mocking me. Growing up, I'd always felt dumb. Testing didn't come easily. I'd see a standardized test with those blank circles staring back at me and would utterly freeze.

"Fill the answers in, A through D. You have one hour," a teacher would say, and the kids around me would look completely unfazed as they scribbled away at their tests while my body shut down at the timed, performative nature of it all. So

I would answer about two questions, freak out about the time, and fill in the rest of the bubbles randomly. I usually finished before everyone and would walk up to hand in my test while the other students' heads were still down, which made me feel freaking fabulous as the kids looked up, undoubtedly assuming I'd aced the test. But then, when my test was returned with a big D– on the front page, I'd be reminded that I was different from other students, and not in a positive way.

So when my therapist said, "You are brilliant," while looking me straight in the eye, I seriously considered telling her to piss off. But instead I listened, and I felt her words shake through me. She continued, "Your body is brilliant because it knows how to survive hard things. It has done what it had to do to adapt, and now it continues to because it is still acting as your protector."

Her words hummed along with the noise machine, a calming cadence that made me feel them like a meditative prayer. I thought about how many times my body's brilliance had shown up over the years, when my hardened skin from scleroderma formed a protective shell over the surface of my body, when my thyroid stopped functioning and highlighted years of voice repression, when my chest became tight and made it difficult to breathe and introduced me to lungs as the home of grief, when my headaches became rampant and revealed the tension I was holding chronically in my neck, when I defaulted to freeze and fawn responses in moments of felt terror, when dissociative spells took over at heightened moments of emotional pain, and so many more.

Alice Miller writes, "Frequently, physical illnesses are the body's response to permanent disregard of its vital functions. One of our most vital functions is an ability to listen to the true story of our own lives."[2] In that therapist's office, for the first time, I believed it. My body was brilliant! My body had held memories, pain, and unspoken stories like forgotten boxes tucked deep in an attic, but now the attic door was flung open. I could see the boxes, and I could touch them. And if I was patient, I could open them carefully, one by one, to see what was inside.

"Your body is brilliant" was perhaps the most validating thing I'd ever heard, and those words marked the beginning of my journey to reframe my body's deep wisdom. From that moment, "being brilliant" wasn't about my scores on a test but a deep trust in my body as my storyteller.

This is why I believe that when we can act as a witness to our own stories, then we can begin to have a conversation with ourselves the way my therapist did with me. We can sit across from the body's narrative and gaze compassionately at the illness and pain, the self-doubt, the internalized shame, and the stories that still sit in silence, waiting for us to turn to them. We can lean toward those brave stories like a good therapist and ask, with empathy, "Do you know how brilliant you are?"

Deep into my study and acceptance of this brilliant body, I dove into the transformational research of author and psychoanalyst Annie Rogers. In her work with young children who had survived sexual violence, she saw that their memory was stored in the subconscious before they had a recollection of what they had experienced. Rogers studied the wordlessness of one young survivor and began to find the truth of the girl's trauma through layers of language, repetition, and the body's speaking. Bit by bit, she helped the young girl find meaning within metaphor and what was rising outside of linear language. She writes in her book *The Unsayable*, "When all the traces of history have been erased and the body itself is inscribed with an unknown language, how does a child begin to speak?"[3]

As I've studied Rogers's stories of young trauma survivors, the stories of women I've worked with, the brilliance of the human body, and my own traversing through stories difficult to name, I've thought about how linear language can be lacking as we explore the tender stories of our past. The alternative route I've found through this fog has been through creative expression, specifically art and poetry, that allow for metaphor and imagery when stories are too difficult to name outright.

This creative expression is a really powerful healing tool, as oftentimes we lose language. Why? Because our bodies hold space for feelings, but words, time, and images can seem muddied. This is why, when we try to talk about difficult events, our words get small, or when we try writing, the details of our memory can be challenging to access.

Not too long ago, I taught a writing workshop titled "Poetry to Heal" that looked at the meaning of metaphor. Perhaps you've seen this, too, in recent works of a poet you love, where they describe grief as a whirlpool they're sinking under or the lack of memory as a crack in the ceiling. What's happening there? They are allowing imagery to speak around an experience that can be hard to describe bluntly. For example, it might be challenging for us to write the outright phrase, "I was abused," but we might be able to write, "My body was filled with gold and they robbed me clean." The gift of poetry allows us to show up to these unsayable words and begin to see them in a different light.

By the end of the workshop, many attendees began to write their silenced stories in verse. They used metaphor and other imagery to release memories in their bodies, intentionally created white space to illustrate blankness and gaps of time, and employed techniques like repetition to highlight a theme. When they stood back from their poetry and read it aloud, they found the unsayable stories tucked inside that they had long forgotten.

For many who have suffered, trauma creates so many complex pieces that integration seems impossible. Our bodies tell us the stories of our trauma, speaking to the fragmentation of mind, body, and spirit through various symptomatic responses. This is why the work of integration and writing from the body is so important. It is an incarnational process, the written word of our lives made flesh.

Trauma does not discriminate; it shows itself in a number of different forms and to any number of people, but its impact is always the same—it shatters us, and healing from it requires a spiritual journey of embodied storytelling, an act of returning home to oneself. We are all writing toward resilience. Every effort we make toward befriending our stories allows for repair where there has been a rupture. So many of us have subconsciously created patterns of self-sabotage over the years, turning unresolved wounds into self-blame. When we write down these wounds, we face off with those old voices and patterns that show up as avoidance, self-doubt, impostor syndrome, and so on. By naming them one at a time, we address the stories that have wounded us over the years so that we can finally write and creatively express ourselves—and be free.

As you explore your unsayable stories and the brilliance of your body, consider how to let words and art flow through you. May the practice of poetry and creative expression help you find the parts that have gone missing and be the next step in your path toward healing and wholeness. After all, Humpty-Dumpty may have missed something. Maybe he wasn't broken beyond repair; maybe, with all those pieces, he could've become a beautiful mosaic.

WRITE ON THIS:

Poetry and Imagery

Our bodies all hold stories, and when we begin to listen to the unsayable, we can uncover their inner wisdom. Often, when stories have been held in our bodies, linear language alone cannot locate them. That is why I recommend poetry or art as another way to explore this telling.

Consider choosing a metaphor for your own body to create a poem from. Think of all the imagery you can pull from this (water, ice, fire, weeds, burial ground, flowers, bones, and so on). Don't forget you can play with white space to communicate your experience as well. Author e. e. cummings was a master at this, by the way, turning the layout of his poetry into something so visually captivating that many could stare at the play of white space and words for hours, his collections moving readers in a way similar to art hung in a gallery.

If writing a poem still feels overwhelming, grab some crayons and a piece of paper and color the feelings in your body. There is no wrong way to do this. Let your inner child arise and make art and poetry without an ounce of critique, just curiosity.

REPEAT AFTER ME

My body is brilliant and is a safe keeper of my stories.

Becoming the Good Samaritan of Your Stories

The Latin word *soma* means *body*, so to engage in somatic writing is to create an embodied writing experience. In the most simplistic description, somatic writing practice invites us to listen to our bodies speak and create from a space of sensory awareness, asking questions like: How does my body feel as I write this sentence? Where do I feel resistance in my body? How can I describe this story with senses that bring it to life? When we do somatic writing, we can allow healing, integration, and wholeness to occur. It can be a powerful healing tool for traumatic experiences, as we often lack language after a painful event.

In some ways, I've been engaging in somatic writing and creativity since I was little, through poems, stories, and intuitive art. I would freewrite, journal, and splatter paint across the walls. Often, what I left on the page or canvas was revelatory, because I didn't know what I knew or felt in my body until it was reflected back to me. This is the power of somatic writing; it can reveal truth within us and materialize what has been internalized.

During a season of deep dissociation, I created a somatic practice that could help me find my feelings outside of talk therapy. It offered a mirror to my emotions that seemed to come only from the unfiltered freedom of creative expression. I covered my entire 650-square-foot apartment with paintings of unprocessed pain, an idea I formed after spending a winter break at an artist's residency. About a dozen other artists and I worked in several mediums and camped out on the studio's open floor. For a week, I hunched over canvas and parchment until my body turned stiff, but I hardly dared to move since the stories of my life began to appear in imagery, one after another. There was no way of knowing what would arrive, and I was a woman possessed by the need to create. I painted stories with acrylic layered with crayon until a memory would arrive and shock me with color.

After that short residency, I returned to my apartment with no more blank canvases to fill up, and yet what I'd produced during my winter break felt like only the tip of the creative iceberg. I needed to make more, so I decided to make my apartment into a canvas. Every wall was painted and scribbled on. Though I was in narrative therapy, words were still lacking when it came to talking about painful events in my life, but in that open room I could freewrite poetry and color my beige walls in currents of red. Most of the time, I didn't know what I was writing or what art would be produced until it was finished. Then, when I stepped back far enough, I could read the words written in black marker or stare into the eyes of a portrait telling me a story I'd forgotten. Though I've paid hundreds of thousands of dollars for therapy and my master's degree in psychology, to this day,

I think my apartment-turned-art-studio is really what set my voice free.

In my artist's apartment, I scribbled a poem on my wall titled "The Guest House" by the Sufi poet Rumi. I wrote it as a reminder to befriend and care for the way trauma was showing up in my body rather than judging or abandoning it. I had carried this essential collection of poetry through every major event of my life—through breakups, dark hours of the soul, lonely train travels across America, and weekly ferry rides across the water to therapy. The pages were scribbled upon, coffee-stained, dog-eared, and painted over. And while there were many poems that revived me from this collection, it was "The Guest House" that I memorized and tattooed to the base of my soul, particularly its opening lines.

> This being human is a guest house.
> Every morning a new arrival.
>
> A joy, a depression, a meanness,
> some momentary awareness comes
> as an unexpected visitor.
>
> Welcome and entertain them all![1]

I loved this poem because it helped me see that my past pain is that "unexpected visitor," bleeding and broken, seeking my attention, knocking at the door of my body. My guests are the wounded children in my dream, the unspoken stories crying out from my body, the sabotage cycles from old fears I'd tried hard to run away from.

Sometimes, when they show up, these guests are also characters from my life I've tried hard to avoid, often wearing garments of shame, anger, and deep sadness. But no matter how many times I've tried to slam the door when they show back up, knocking, my most profound healing has come when I've finally opened the door to all the parts of my stories I've been afraid to know.

I grew up hearing the parable of the good Samaritan shared from the pulpit at least once or twice a year. It's a story that had everyone turning their pockets inside out for strangers on the street after an inspiring service, but rarely, if ever, did it make us consider looking at the stranger within ourselves. In this parable, we're told,

> This fellow was traveling down from Jerusalem to Jericho when some robbers mugged him. They took his clothes, beat him to a pulp, and left him naked and bleeding and in critical condition. By chance, a priest was going down that same road, and when he saw the wounded man, he crossed over to the other side and passed by. Then a Levite who was on his way to assist in the temple also came and saw the victim lying there, and he too kept his distance. Then a despised Samaritan journeyed by. When he saw the fellow, he felt compassion for him. The Samaritan went over to him, stopped the bleeding, applied some first aid, and put the poor fellow on his donkey. He brought the man to an inn and cared for him through the night.[2]

Like those who passed by the wounded man on the road, so often we pass by our own painful stories. We neglect what has already been neglected and curse our own body's experience. It makes sense, after all, that this cursing or abandonment of ourselves can sometimes feel easier than blessing our desire for hope and care from another. Can we bless our enemies—that is, the felt opposition deep inside our own skin? Can we pray for that which persecutes us—the physical symptoms, heartache, and reminders of a grief we've tried hard to avoid? When we listen for the breath of our soma narratives, pay attention to cries of abandonment, and know grief in the presence of a witness, we can choose blessing, not cursing; life, not death.

This somatic narrative can feel intrusive, as though it is knocking from the inside of us. It asks of us boldly—Will we answer? This guest is bleeding and broken, seeking our attention—Will we care for them? This guest is us, the many unspoken stories that often feel like a stranger we should avoid. If we answer the door, we welcome the parts of our stories we've been afraid to know. If we invite them in, we invite the hospitality of ourselves despite our hesitation. If we touch them, we touch the parts of ourselves we've cut off and abandoned. Here, the unwelcome guest invites us to heal ourselves by being the good Samaritan of our own story.

After a year, it was time to leave my artist's apartment. That meant painting over the giant canvas that had helped me heal my stories. It took three coats before the art stopped showing through. (And no, in case you were wondering, I definitely did not get my deposit back from my landlord.) I remember a friend saying at the time, "Megan, aren't you sad to paint over your walls?" But I wasn't. I wasn't sad at all. I was relieved at the catharsis it created in me—letting it go, being free of it. Just as painting the space was about getting the pain out of my body, painting over it was symbolic too. I was releasing it.

I repeatedly return to this parable of the good Samaritan because it reminds me to be the Samaritan of my own abandoned stories. When "unwelcome guests" show up at my door dressed in the past, and I'm afraid to confront them, the parable asks me, *Will you recognize them? Will you hear the cry? Will you care for that wounded stranger, or will you continue to pass them by like the priest and the Levite, even though your stories wail from your insides?*

Here is what I know now: when the stories are summoned to the surface, when the blank pages of our lives stare back at us, waiting for us to engage them, when the old narratives show up as guests we are hesitant to be a good Samaritan for, we must turn toward and not away from them. When our bodies speak, and we listen to them, we take the spiritual road of healing through kindness, care, and creative compassion. Learning to welcome the stranger within me and becoming the good Samaritan of my own story has changed my life.

Think about this for yourself. What would it mean to let your body write and create for you? What would it feel like to let go and witness yourself with kindness and compassion? What trust would be created in your body's experience when self-contempt converts to self-love?

The first step to creating a somatic writing practice is to have compassion for yourself—to release the pressure of being "good enough" and let whatever needs to flow through you just flow. Trying to force word counts and ideas to a page can often trigger a feeling of entrapment, similar to past trauma. As you begin to create your own somatic writing practice, consider how to let words and art flow through you.

The second step is to give yourself permission to create from your subconscious without judgment or expectation. This allowance will create trust in your body and mind toward your creative output. Often, we need to restore trust in our writing because we have been so harsh about what we've produced in the past.

Lastly, the third step is to treat this somatic practice as a meditation. When we listen to our bodies, breathe deeply, and pause as we need to, we create a resilient relationship with our story healing and our somatic experience as we hold space for our inner voices to emerge.

WRITE ON THIS:

A New Samaritan Story

It is a powerful reframe to view our stories from the lens of the good Samaritan parable. It can change how we show up to the wounds of our lives. Consider how you have or have not been a good Samaritan to your stories and writing so far. In what ways could you begin to bring better hospitality, wound care, compassion, and empathy into your own stories of somatic healing? Try writing a new Samaritan story for yourself as both the wounded person and the advocate inviting them to heal.

REPEAT AFTER ME

*I am offering hospitality
to all the parts of my stories.*

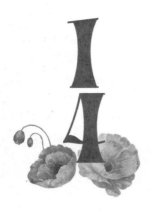

Writing Through Attachment Styles

In my North Louisiana neighborhood, the ditches were like urban swamps muddled with green slime and dirty water. They were mostly underground culverts but surfaced in some surprising places—the back alley behind some of my friends' houses, the dead ends of streets that people avoided altogether, and next to parks where children would play on swings and jungle gyms. They were created to prevent flooding when the storms came through, and a hard rain would fill them up in a minute. The ditches weren't just holding rainwater, though, but often sewage, trash, and even high levels of methamphetamines. We didn't care and didn't even know what these things were or meant; we just knew we were told not to play by the ditches—and so we did.

I spent a lot of time in those ditches back then, especially in the summer season when they were dry, and I would crawl through to see how far I could go before the light at the opening would fade away. I liked the damp smell, the cold concrete, the darkness with a hint of light bursting through the opening. When I didn't go exploring on my own, I went with my brothers on local adventures where the ditches were deeper and wider than the ones I found for myself. We would crawl deep inside their mouths with tiny flashlights as we played hide-and-seek and hunted snapping turtles. Yet when the thunder started miles away, we made sure to crawl out before the storm clouds turned dark overhead. That is because on rainy days, the ditches would fill up fast, drowning many a kid who got stuck in the flash flood.

My brothers were the brave ones, carrying the giant turtles back to our house to keep as newfound pets. One of them would hold either side of the big shell while its slimy green legs hung loosely from its body. Then he'd set it in a laundry basket on an old pink towel, and we'd watch that turtle sit there, still as could be, head buried deep in its shell as if trying to decide whether it was safe to stretch its neck out and survey its new, strange surroundings.

We would name them, usually something from *Teenage Mutant Ninja Turtles* like Michelangelo or Leonardo, giving them funny voices and personalities like what we'd heard on TV. Every once in a while, when I'd start calling to them, the turtle would poke its head out, its mouth sharp like a bird's beak.

"Don't you put your hand close, or it'll bite your finger off!" Momma would yell at us from across the house, and sure enough, I nearly got bit a couple of times when my brothers dared me to pet it on the places where the skin was soft. I loved the complexity of these creatures, with the shell of their outer body hard like armor, thick and protective, and yet their soft underbelly smooth like butter, the very epitome of vulnerability.

After a few hours and Momma's hollering to get that turtle out of the kitchen, one or the other of my brothers would take the snapping turtle back to the ditch to set it free. He would set it down on the swampy concrete, gently ushering it back to where it came from. Yet the turtle would usually just stand there awkwardly, frozen from fear that it might get snatched up again. I didn't blame it; I would've been scared too.

As I reflect on it now, I can see that those turtles and I were made of the same stuff, at least metaphorically—I, too, had a hard shell on the outside but was soft and tender in the places harder to see. I struggled to get close to people while feeling guarded and fearful of what could happen if I let others in. I watched my peers become close with seeming ease at a young age and even participate in each other's weddings decades later, yet I had difficulty remaining in close contact with anyone I knew from childhood. It was more natural for me to stay in my turtle shell and poke my head out only when it felt safe.

When I began to write stories about my life, and especially when I shared myself publicly, I felt that vulnerability even more, as though my outer shell had been taken completely off and my underbelly was exposed to the world. It felt dangerous and utterly stupid—why write hard things that could hurt me? But there was something in me that said *It hurts more to hold it in*. So I persevered. And with each act of sharing, I sensed a new kind of protection forming, not a hard outer shield but something within me that strengthened every time I took a risk and used my voice.

The understanding that came from writing down the hard stuff made me think about those summer days in the ditch. Those snapping turtles were teaching me early on about the transformation that comes from the risk of vulnerability but also teaching me the importance of boundaries set to guard our hearts against those who could hurt us. Over the years, I've learned that it's really about the balance of both—the tender and the tough. Our loving, hoping, and story healing must exist somewhere between the two. We can have a thick exterior in confronting the past and a soft underbelly to let ourselves be known for who we are.

I can always tell I am onto something important when my turtle shell reappears, and I become avoidant. My old anxious attachment style kicks in, and I begin playing hide-and-seek again, hiding behind busyness, brainstorming, new projects—anything, really—to keep from showing up to my stories. When resistance shows up in all of its avoidance, we can know we are being called to write the thing we're most afraid of. As Steven Pressfield writes in *The War of Art*, "Are you paralyzed with fear? That's a good sign. Fear is good. Like self-doubt, fear is an indicator. Fear tells us what we have to do. Remember our rule of thumb: the more scared we are of a work or calling, the more sure we can be that we have to do it."[1] The resistance is here to teach us, working like an alarm, highlighting our old attachment wounds that have been left unresolved.

I first came to the language of attachment theory around the time I first entered the Womb Room and felt the familiar fear of being seen, known, and loved in a room full of people. It was a fear I'd felt for as long as I could remember. I'd always struggled to initiate the phrase "I love you" to family or others close to me. I was even nicknamed "Side Hugger" by my friends because all my hugs were given from a distance with a quick three taps on the back as if to say, "Okay, that's enough. Goodbye for now."

The thing is, we are created for attachment, to be in union and not in isolation. From the moment we are born, we cry out for the safety of another womb. We have an intrinsic longing to be contained, wrapped, and fed. The theory of attachment was developed to observe and study this early need for connection, specifically in the parent-child relationship. Through these studies, theorists have identified four styles of attachment: secure, anxious-avoidant, fearful-ambivalent, and disorganized.[2] Each child's reactions to moments of separation and return with their caregiver show how that child perceives relational connection with the world around them.

One famous study of these styles was "The Strange Situation," created by researcher Mary Ainsworth. It looked at mother-child relationships and how infants reacted to proximity, separation, and return. In this space, Ainsworth integrated a short drama that tested the child's reactions to their mother's departure and return while bringing a stranger into the room to interact with the child between these moments.

Through this study, Ainsworth concluded that it was the infant's responses to the reunion rather than the separation that spoke volumes. What she found was that a securely attached infant would be distressed by separation yet mostly reassured when the mother returned to the room. An insecure-avoidant child would adopt a passive and dismissive attitude. A fearful-avoidant child would be distressed by the unpredictability of when or if the mother would return at all, often becoming angry and inconsolable. And lastly, the disorganized child would be caught in a web of emotional chaos, filled with the uncertainty of whether the mother was safe or sometimes to be feared upon her return.[3]

From this attachment theory, a concept called the "good-enough mother" emerged.[4] This idea is that a person can develop a secure attachment style if they are in a safe and consistent environment of relational care over time. Discovering this made me think about how our own stories can serve as the "good-enough mother," offering the stability we need through mirroring and reflecting our truth.

How might our story healing evolve if we viewed it through the lens of attachment theory? If you consider each attachment style and how it might show up in your story work, through that awareness you can begin taking steps to build a secure relationship with your stories. I have personally seen myself a bit in all of the attachment styles; maybe you will too. Let's break them down to see how each style might show up when we're writing.

First, the *insecure-avoidant storyteller*, at their core, is fearful of abandonment and rejection. They believe everyone else has something important and relevant to say, but their own story is insignificant in comparison. They may write a story they deeply believe in but minimize its power or description to avoid someone not accepting it as good enough. Ultimately, they have created an island within themselves to protect them from future loss, even if that loss never shows up.

For the insecure-avoidant storyteller, *hope* is a bad word, and it is a dangerous risk to trust that their voice has power. Their story process highlights their attachment wound through impostor syndrome and the devaluation of their voice. When they say about their story, "It isn't that interesting," or "Others have more to say than me," I ask them if they are willing to say these same words to their younger self.

There is no hesitation in their response: "Absolutely not."

As we sit across from one another, I tell them how proud I am that they are being honest with themselves and with me about how they truly feel. Slowly, they begin to show up to their stories with the attention and care of a "good mother." Their journey toward healing this attachment wound may look like applying affirmations with the words they write, finding ongoing encouragement that their voice matters, and practicing trust in the process as they inch toward security.

Next, the *fearful-ambivalent storyteller* may feel terrified to commit to a story or complete a creative project fully. They try to reconcile this fear by staying busy, juggling a million possibilities to avoid the potential of hurt that may or may not ever come. The irony is that they crave consistency and yet perpetuate distraction to avoid what they fear most. The steps they are called to take in working with this fear are to try focusing their attention on one story at a time, feeling the feelings that arise, and staying with themselves until they arrive at some ending. In doing this, they become the good mother who stays in moments of stress when writing their stories.

In a coaching call, I listen to the same storyteller share how they can't seem to complete the book that has been on their heart for years. "I just keep getting distracted by other things. I guess I am scared of what will happen if I finish it. Will I succeed, or will I fail?" They hold the weight of these possibilities, both equally terrifying. I understand how much more comfortable it is to stay ambivalent rather than make a choice. I know this fear well in my body as I say to them, "I juggle a lot of things at once, too, because I am afraid of the responsibility that comes with completing something." Then we make a plan together to focus on one thing at a time, with approachable markers in place for predictability, and we set up honesty emails with one another to express how we feel rather than keeping it inside. Bit by bit, I see this writer find stability in their storytelling when they complete one chapter after another, practicing accepting and forgiving themselves along the way.

Last, *the disorganized storyteller* will feel torn between finding writing to be a place of safety and yet simultaneously a source of fear. They are tossed between the longing to create and the anticipation that if they take the risk, something bad waits on the other side. This causes a current of inconsistency in their writing process. One day they are inspired and the next distrustful. The next day they are determined to show up, but the following day finds them running away from the project as fast as they can.

One disorganized storyteller I worked with wanted to write their trauma story because they were trying to gather all the pieces of their life and make sense of the past. They began with incredible hope and expectation, plowing ahead in their writing with a fervor I couldn't begin to keep up with. Then, after a short time, they hit a brick wall from burnout. They had pushed beyond their emotional readiness and entered into a place of retraumatization. The story they felt empowered and excited to tell became a trigger, replicating past pain. "I can't write anymore. It hurts too much," they told me with tears in their eyes. I held the space for them and listened in silence. I didn't want to fill up the room with a response; I wanted this storyteller to fill it up with their truth. They were caught in the paradox of feeling both safety and debilitating fear in their writing at the same time.

After a few minutes, they said, "I want to write, but I want to go slow and take care of myself along the way." Together, we created a trauma-informed plan for how to listen, care, and pace themselves in the process. They would return to the old attachment room where their earliest wounds resided and sit with them in stillness. Little by little, sharing with people who are safe listeners and creating stability for their writing process will help them feel grounded and held.

All three of these storytellers are making their way toward a *secure attachment*, one in which they feel safe to express themselves, safe to complete a project, and safe to take their time in the telling. Through their story healing, they are learning to be the good mother with their bounty of words as well as the absence of them, all without judgment. This "good mother" is the epitome of compassion and presence in our storytelling and is key in cultivating a secure attachment with our sacred stories.

One of my favorite quotes of all time that represents this so well is by Annie Dillard in *The Writing Life*, where she illustrates this compassionate, secure attachment in our writing: "I do not so much write a book as sit up with it, as with a dying friend. During visiting hours, I enter its room with dread and sympathy for its many disorders. I hold its hand and hope it will get better."[5] Every time I read this, I cry. I cry because when we can come to our stories with this kind of compassion, when we can dare to remove our protective turtle shells in vulnerability and show up to grieve our abandoned stories, then we can begin to repair the old, ruptured attachment wounds of our past and reparent our brave stories.

We can create a secure attachment every time we show up, listen, and stay present with our stories when everything within us wants to run away. This act of presence is the work of resilience as we grow to embrace the both/and—the toughness of a turtle shell created by good boundaries and self-care as well as the tenderness of soft skin that is moved by vulnerability. May we all continue to heal through the practice of being the good mother as we reparent our stories into a secure attachment that allows them to feel safe in the holding.

WRITE ON THIS:

Secure Attachment

Consider the four attachment styles: anxious/avoidant, fearful/ambivalent, disorganized, and secure. When we have wisdom around how each of these appears in our lives and our personal writing, we can begin to practice secure attachment by being the "good mother" in our own story healing.

Reflect on what that secure attachment looks like for you. Perhaps it is showing patience, choosing kindness over contempt, creating safe spaces to share your stories with another, or something similar. Then write a short letter to yourself about how you want to create security with your words and stories. Put this letter somewhere close by as a reminder to cultivate care.

REPEAT AFTER ME

I am healing the attachment wounds of my stories and creating safety and security for my voice.

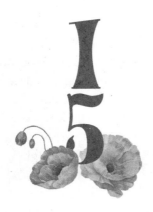

Rebuilding After
the Rupture

Within attachment theory is a concept created by John Bowlby known as relational rupture and repair,[1] which speaks to the breaking and mending process that happens within relationships from an early age. These ruptures, whether big or small, are inevitable in our lives, but by offering these ruptures repair, we can create new routes toward resilience, which is so essential to healing the cracks within our stories.

Growing up in Louisiana, I learned about ruptures early on from how the land would flood so easily because it was below sea level. It was not uncommon for the streets to fill and overflow onto the sidewalks. On super stormy days in New Orleans, a downpour could cover the entire city in minutes.

I remember one year when the city flooded multiple times. We could tell when it was going to be a flood day because we'd receive a familiar ping on our phones, a warning message from the city: "Move your vehicles to high land. High probability of flooding." And so cars started lining up on the slightly elevated Lafitte Greenway in hopes that they wouldn't wash away. This didn't always work, and depending on how much rain fell and how quickly, some cars would just be picked up by the water like they weighed nothing at all. If you haven't lived in New Orleans, it might sound strange, but this was a pretty normal occurrence. Yes, it is stressful, but the magical city is worth it; that said, you better have some really rad car insurance.

During one of these downpours, Landon and I were out listening to the music at a nearby jazz club. There was no time to drive back to our house before the streets flooded, so we parked in the most elevated place we could find and prayed our lowrider Cadillac could stay above water until the storm subsided. Then we ran back home, raindrops as big as pennies hitting our faces. In less than fifteen minutes, the water was up to our knees, and residents had already started pulling out their kayaks to ride the Venice-like streets. We trudged through the swamped city, manically laughing as neighbors waved from boats as we passed by.

The next day, we returned to get our car. It was as though it had all been a dream. Nothing looked out of the ordinary; the streets were dry, the kayaks were put up, and cars moved along the roads just fine. Other than a couple of vehicles left stranded and flooded beyond repair, everything looked completely normal, like there hadn't just been a flash flood that ruptured everyday life.

This polarity felt familiar. The highs of spontaneous parade celebrations and dancing in the jazz-filled streets and the lows of uncertainty that came with the deluges reminded me of the grief that lived within me—the kind I could feel rising like sewer water but that, on the outside, no one could see. Like those flash floods that appeared out of nowhere, so was the grief and sadness that sat below sea level, leaving my body soaked through with vulnerability caused by the emotional wounds that came through my story healing. Their tide would make the water climb far past my ankles, but somehow I wouldn't fall over.

I think of these flood days often when I begin to feel the rupture of old stories and the necessary repair that must come in healing them. I realize now that these have been some of my biggest teachers in story healing. They remind me to swim deep but not so far that the depths prove dangerous. Just like we park our cars on high land to keep them from flooding, we write through our stories and healing process from a safe and observant place. I anchor into the assurance that uncovering stories and past pain is like the grief water rising yet also our life preserver as we reflect, write, and steady ourselves into the reminder that though the waters rise, they also subside.

I recall the summer Hurricane Katrina hit, and the devastation showed up in a way no one anticipated. I joined a disaster relief team, and we went into districts where the levees had broken and the flooding had just consumed houses. Neighborhoods that had once been bustling with life—music on porches, kids running the streets, gardening in the front yards—were now like graveyards. Still and completely silent.

We focused on one house at a time. Many had to be gutted to the studs to see where rebuilding could begin. It was strange to see what was once a home so emaciated, all the walls removed and only the foundation and wood beams left. Sometimes the family would be there, and we would work alongside them, searching for anything that might be salvageable from the rupture of the sudden storm.

One house stands out in my memory. I was digging through piles of debris, and I came across a family photo album. How it was untouched is still a miracle to me. I carried the album outside to the homeowners, whose faces were sagging with the weight of grief as they carried parts of their house to the side of the street. As I handed this couple their album, their faces changed, and another levee broke—but this time within their bodies as they cried, clutching the album with one hand and each other with the other. I remember their words well: "This is literally all we have left now."

After that long day, I walked down the street to get some air free of the smell of mold and wet insulation. I needed to let myself cry for these families that felt the violence of the storm. I looked around the neighborhood; the search and rescue teams had marked the doors with red Xs, and it looked like a zombie town. I stepped over cracks in the road formed from a land sinking from too much precipitation. But in one of those cracks, there was a tiny bit of evidence of repair. There, within the divide in the concrete, a flower had started to bloom in a place that seemed to have little opportunity for life. And yet, there it was: God existing in the cracks where people often forget to look.

I couldn't help but think about the impact of trauma that hits like a hurricane, how it tears through the whole house of us, leaving not much but debris—except for maybe that one album or that one tiny flower. It is a small semblance of hope that comes in the form of a question: Where do you begin to rebuild when the heaps of rubble are twice your size, and all you have is a measly shovel? One scoop at a time, one wall at a time, you clear out the old so you can make room for the new.

There are some ruptures in our stories that come like a hurricane and can make us feel washed away by the emotional torrents, leaving only pieces of a life left behind. Still, there are also many moments of repair in which we can show up to these stories, witness their catastrophic effects, and begin rebuilding from the foundation up.

I liken this story repair process to disaster relief work. We show up at the affected site, evaluate the scene, and make a plan for repair based on the severity of the devastation. We put on our safety gear: gloves and boots to avoid exposed nails and insulation, masks to prevent inhalation of mold, and goggles for flying debris. Then we begin excavating the parts of the house that are no longer salvageable, such as furniture, walls, and carpets. We remove what was necessary so that we can rebuild the home with brand-new materials.

We can show up to our wounded stories the same way. We can look honestly at how each rupture occurred and the impact it has made on our lives. Then we make a plan for addressing our wounded stories with safety for ourselves in the process and care for what is being excavated from within. When we have sat with the houses of our stories—the structure, the ruptures, and the repair—then we can begin to rebuild narratives one brick at a time with an awareness of the past, safety for the present, and an embodied process for a future that continues to unfold.

WRITE ON THIS:

Rupture and Repair

Consider a time when you experienced a rupture; perhaps it was an emotional wound, a heartbreak, or a sudden loss. When you think about that rupture, how did it impact you and your trust in the world? Then, consider what it might look like to repair and rebuild what was broken. If you have a repair story for that rupture, write it down. If it is something you are still in the devastation of, write the repair you long for.

For example, I may recall the devastation from the assault I experienced. I approach the story with honesty. I write it with safety and self-care. Then, I reflect on the repair that has happened since that moment and the repair that continues to unfold—like an understanding of my body's trauma response, compassion for my choices in a devastating betrayal, and gratitude for my ongoing journey of trust in myself and others.

There is powerful healing that comes in acknowledging the rupture and powerful transformation that follows with the repair. Enter the foundations of your stories with kindness, compassion, and care. Your stories are holding you, and you are holding them.

REPEAT AFTER ME

I am more than the ruptures of my past. I am repairing a future for my stories.

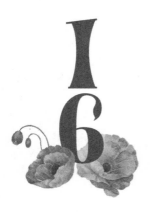

We Can't Outrun
Our Stories

The first ten years of our marriage, Landon and I moved more than ten times! Usually, I was the one to prompt it when my body became restless and the old familiar *stuckness* settled in. Just a few months after our wedding, we were renting a place in north Seattle. I remembered one day there in particular, when my wife-body was standing over a stove making salmon and sweet potatoes. I was freshly unemployed, wearing a domestic uniform of womanly house duties I didn't recognize myself in. I felt lost, insecure, and most of all, bored.

We fought a lot back then. These were manic explosions, usually after too much alcohol, that resulted in me literally running away when the conversation got too hard. Once I left Landon in the parked car with the engine still on and ran for blocks in a drunken haze. My feet pounded the hard concrete until I was nearly a mile away. Then, out of breath and out of places to run to, I stumbled back to the house. After these explosions we would fall back into each other's arms and cover our bodies with apology.

In truth? I was afraid I was going to fade away in that wife-body, that endless existential crisis, that futile searching for self. I felt like a boat lost at sea in my new role and had zero sense of direction. I didn't know that having a partnership would be a new kind of transition into healing my stories.

It was a difficult road that would ask me to keep looking inward, but from a vantage point of safe attachment instead of the broken ones of my past. When I fell in love, I'd naively expected that somehow it would help me bypass the pain I'd avoided. Still, like all things true and transformational, our stories will continue digging away at the outward barriers we've created to keep from trusting ourselves. One after another they fall, until we reach the core of who we are becoming.

One year into our marriage, we proposed a move to New York City. It was probably said as a joke, but I took it in truth, packed up my bags, and was ready to go. We sold everything except for what we could fit into a rental van and drove across the country. As we traveled through one state after another, I looked at Landon, afraid. "What if we leave and start over, but this vacancy follows me there? What if this isn't about where we go? What if it's deeper? What if it is within me?" I asked.

Not long after we arrived, I stood in the bustle of a subway station, surrounded by bodies of strangers all moving from one place to another. I felt small in the midst of them, but even still, I began going out on my own, getting lost, panicking, and then doing it all over again.

I explored museums alive with art and stopped to listen to musicians whose voices echoed across the tunnel walls. I took on jobs that stretched me beyond my comfort zone, jobs I never thought I could do beforehand but in that moment felt possible in my new skin. I visited human trafficking shelters where I'd sit with women and help them tell their stories, stories that helped me see human resilience in a whole new light. I taught yoga at corporate offices in Rockefeller Center to men in Armani suits who sat across from me as I taught their busy bodies to breathe in the midst of chaos. I hosted storytelling events at some of the famous venues in town where musical heroes of mine, like Patti Smith and David Byrne, had once graced the same stages I now stood on.

I shook in these spaces, too, just like I had when the spotlight shone down on me during my first solo in elementary school, but with every decision I made that scared me there also came new confidence. Each was a rite of passage from being a woman uncertain of herself to a woman unafraid to be fully in her body.

On one cold winter morning, I took a walk on the edge of Greenpoint. The wind chill off the East River was -2 degrees, making my cheeks prick and sting. I wrapped my scarf up to my nose, eyes wet from the cold as I took in the smog that hovered over the Hudson River, blurring the tall buildings in the distance. The questions returned that I'd asked Landon on our move to New York: *What if I leave and this sadness follows me there? What if it is within me?* I had an answer now: yes. It had followed me, but this time, I wasn't afraid to be with the feeling. Over the soft swell of the river, the words that had been hot on my heels for years finally caught up to me: *You can't outrun your stories.* With them came a sense of resolve. I could finally rest in the reality that I could stop running if I wanted to.

I had felt this statement when I splashed into the Atlantic at age six, when my brother tore up the letter I wrote him after I slid it under his door, when I searched for story healing that launched me into graduate school. It was the same statement that told me to paint on a canvas and put words on a page. *You can't outrun the stories within you, no matter how many times you try to avoid them.*

All the journeying, the hiding, the transitioning was not so much about the external as it was the internal. There had been movement happening in me for years, wandering from one dislocated part of myself to another, leaving me exhausted. And each transition just seemed to pronounce this sense of inner ache, a longing to live a full, truthful, and thriving story. When I finally stopped the search from outside of me and began to look within, I was terrified, if I'm being real, and it broke me into pieces. But it also made me the artist that I am—collaging memory, weaving metaphor into verse, making art out of forgotten things.

When we experience loss in our lives—a person, a dream, an evolution of faith—it becomes increasingly difficult to connect with our passions, desires, and longings. Why? We internalize the loss as betrayal and regret. "If only I hadn't hoped for so much. . . . If only I hadn't let my guard down. . . . If only I hadn't put my heart out there." The desire that was once beautiful and full of wonder transforms into this dangerous thing we resent ourselves for having. Thus, we keep moving, stay busy, and live our lives in a restless spree of distraction. But in the words of thirteenth-century mystic Meister Eckhart, "Spirituality is not to be learned by flight from the world, or by running away from things, or by turning solitary and going apart from the world. Rather, we must learn an inner solitude wherever or with whomsoever we may be."[1]

This is why we must reconcile with the parts of our stories we've exiled. We must stay with the pieces of ourselves we've kept abandoning. When we do this work of paying attention and *staying* amid life's many transitions, then we will know the true meaning of home. The word *transition* comes from the Latin for "go across," but go across what? For each person, those crossings will look and feel different and take more or less time. For me, many of my crossings have looked familiar, like roads I'd been on in the past but hadn't returned to in years. Part of my work in transition is to slow down, take in the scenery of past and present, and let myself stop along the way to forgive, reconcile, and plant seeds of resilience.

The beautiful invitation of story healing is to embrace the many transitions you go through in your journey, honor your nomadic spirit, reconcile with any part of yourself you've run away from, and practice the art of staying true to whatever crossing you're at.

This work of knowing our bodies as storytellers and bandaging the wounds of the pages of our lives is not a one-stop shop; it is a spiritual progression. As we heal our lives, brave the page, and continue the curious and compassionate work of listening and loving our narratives, we will begin to gather our many pieces into our whole selves, becoming the advocates our stories have always needed.

A Blessing for Your Ever-Evolving Story

I bless this season of transition
May this disruption be beautiful,
and an awakening for the evolution of you

I bless who you are becoming
May all that you have learned over the years
continue to shape your soul toward love and kindness

I bless your creativity and longing
May your desire to create be met with
devotion to the divine calling within you

I bless the resistance you feel toward your stories
May the places that feel stuck and blocked
be opened and cleared for expression

I bless the void, the formlessness, the darkness in
   Genesis stories
May the blankness you feel lead you always
on a nomadic journey toward compassion and
   self-care

I bless the ache in you for a whole story
May all parts of you be met with curiosity
As you become the glorious mosaic you were always
   meant to be

WRITE ON THIS:
Closing Reflection

As a closing reflection, consider the various transitions your life has invited you to. What crossings have been most transformational for you? Write them down as stories and poems that you can look back on as part of your journey. When you finish, piece these writings together like pearls strung onto a necklace.

I am reconciling with the parts of my stories I've exiled. I am coming home to myself.

CLOSING THOUGHTS

You have reached the end of this book but not the end of your stories. I hope it has offered illuminations for your life and given you a glimpse of how braving the page and expressing yourself creatively can unlock the stories your body holds. Know this: You are the healer of your own stories. You have everything within you to unwrap your truth and awaken your desire. The hardest part is remaining open to listening and continuing to show up to hear your life speak. As psychologist Judith Herman writes, "The first principle of recovery is empowerment of the survivor. She must be the author and arbiter of her own recovery. Others may offer advice, support, assistance, affection, and care, but not cure."[1]

Healing our stories is a lifelong journey we continue throughout our lives. The gift it offers us is one we will always be unwrapping. As I've mentioned throughout, story healing has nothing to do with identifying as a writer or creative; it is about the practice of paying attention to the stories within and digging into the deep questions that our stories ask of us. Writing and creative expression just happen to be the radical tools that help us cultivate curiosity for our own sacred stories.

I hope that as you reflect on the words in this book, they serve as a catalyst for your healing. May this book be dog-eared and highlighted, may its pages be torn out and posted as reminders, and may its edges be filled with your own brave reflections.

Here are a few reminders to take with you on the road:

1. Healing is not a linear process. There is no point A and point B. You must allow yourself to shift, move, fall, and grow, all in the name of process.
2. You can't rush your healing. It takes time, and that's okay. Give yourself grace and compassion to feel all that you need at the pace that you need.
3. You don't have to do this alone. Trauma recovery can feel so isolating. You need people and communities you can trust to share your voice and story with.
4. Brave the page. Show up to regular writing and creative practice as a way to listen to your life. This is not about writing well and making "good" art. This is about the beautiful process of creative writing and what it will teach you along the way.
5. Practice creative consensuality in your story healing. The more you remind yourself that you have choice and agency in your voice, the less burnout and emotional exhaustion you will face as you navigate stories.
6. Safety is paramount. As you enter your journey toward deeper story work, remember to find your edges and practice self-care such as breathwork, embodied awareness, and taking necessary pauses to prioritize your mental health. If you have access to a support group or a counselor to process with, that could be a safe space as well.

7. You are growing in resilience. Just as story healing is ongoing, so is your resilience developing as you face the ruptures and practice repair through writing and reflection.

8. Your body holds stories. Sometimes you can't say how you feel, but your body can clue you in. Listen to your body with open ears. Consider the story your body is trying to tell you.

9. Thank yourself often. There is power in gratitude. When you show up to your stories, you are doing the work of an advocate in caring, listening, and providing safe support. Acknowledge the holding space within you that is helping you heal.

10. Stay kind. You're fighting a hard battle. You have made it this far, and you will make it even further. You are loved, and you are not alone as you keep going.

ACKNOWLEDGMENTS

Thank you to my agent, Morgan, for your belief in my voice and your fierce advocacy to get it into the hands of the perfect editor and publisher for this work. I didn't realize how much I longed for an ally in this writing process until you came along. You are a blessing.

Thank you to my editors Stephanie and Grace, as well as the entire team at Baker Books, for seeing the importance of this book and believing in the importance of writing to heal. Stephanie, your wisdom and eyes on this project have challenged me to show up with more honesty, clarity, and deep trust in my voice. I am in awe of your love for words and your ability to see beyond the curtain.

Thank you to the hundreds of writing clients I have had the privilege of working with. Your bravery in showing up to your stories and taking the risk to write what you are called to has impacted me more than words can say. You are my inspiration for getting honest, writing with care and compassion, and going for what you long for with a fierce determination. May all your writing dreams come true!

Thank you to Dan Allender and The Seattle School. Your wisdom and mentorship in my own story healing have been some of the biggest catalysts in my life. I am forever grateful to you for holding the torch through the dark days of my discovery.

Thank you to my family and to Louisiana, which shaped so much of my stories. From the bumpy road trips to the music that rang through our home, to deep conversations that were both rocky and beautiful, to magnolia trees and thunderstorms that kept me up at night, and of course, to all the crayfish boils. I am forever grateful for the teachings that have come through you all.

Thank you to all the friends who celebrated every little writing win with flowers and celebratory dinners and who sent texts that cheered me on when I thought I was done. Your kindness kept me afloat, even if you had no idea I needed it. I love you.

Thank you to the mystery of God in the light, the shadow, and the darkness. We have wrestled hard, Lord, and yet I've found you let me linger in the hard questions without answers, and I love you for that. May our conversations continue always and be filled with the risk to hope.

Lastly, thank you to my Landon, who has endlessly supported my creativity and writing journey. You have listened to me read chapter after chapter with such an open heart and have offered wisdom that has made me a better and more honest writer. I truly don't know where I'd be without your fierce love and friendship in my life. I love you, babe.

NOTES

Hello, Body

1. Gabor Maté, *When the Body Says No: Exploring the Stress-Disease Connection* (John Wiley & Sons, 2003), 2.

2. Maté, *When the Body Says No*, 3, 2.

3. Caroline Myss, *Anatomy of the Spirit: The Seven Stages of Power and Healing* (Harmony, 1996), 40.

4. Mary Oliver, "The Uses of Sorrow," *Thirst: Poems* (Beacon Press, 2006), 52.

5. Franz Kafka, "Letter to Oskar Pollak, January 27, 1904," in *Letters to Friends, Family, and Editors*, 3rd ed., trans. Richard Winston and Clara Winston (Schocken Books, 2016), 16.

6. Annie G. Rogers, *The Unsayable: The Hidden Language of Trauma* (Ballantine Books, 2007).

7. See Ezekiel 37:1–14.

Chapter 1 Collecting Memories

1. Anne Lamott, *Bird by Bird: Some Instructions on Writing and Life*, 25th anniv. ed. (Anchor Books, 2019), 4.

2. Lynda Barry, *Making Comics* (Drawn and Quarterly, 2019), 3.

3. As quoted in Bryce Nelson, "Why Are Earliest Memories So Fragmented and Elusive?" *New York Times*, December 7, 1982, https://www.ny times.com/1982/12/07/science/why-are-earliest-memories-so-fragmentary -and-elusive.html.

4. "Paresthesia," Cleveland Clinic, accessed May 7, 2024, https://my.cleve landclinic.org/health/symptoms/24932-paresthesia.

5. Joy Harjo, "For Calling the Spirit Back from Wandering the Earth in Its Human Feet," in *Conflict Resolution for Holy Beings: Poems* (W. W. Norton, 2015), 6.

6. Jodi Picoult, *Handle with Care: A Novel* (Washington Square Press, 2009), 435.

7. As quoted in Nelson, "Why Are Earliest Memories So Fragmentary and Elusive?"

Chapter 2 The Power of Genesis Stories

1. Kendra Cherry, "What Is the Negativity Bias?" Verywell Mind, November 13, 2023, https://www.verywellmind.com/negative-bias-4589618.

2. Genesis 1:1–2 NKJV.

3. As quoted in Jia Tolentino, "Hall of Mirrors," *Slate*, March 3, 2015, https://slate.com/culture/2015/03/ongoingness-by-sarah-manguso-reviewed.html.

4. Steve Madigan, "Narrative Therapy: Deconstructing & Re-Authoring Stories," Counseling Education, accessed May 10, 2024, https://counseling.education/counseling/theories/narrative.html.

5. Chimamanda Ngozi Adichie, "The Danger of a Single Story," TED Talk, TEDGlobal 2009, accessed July 31, 2024, https://www.ted.com/talks/chimamanda_ngozi_adichie_the_danger_of_a_single_story?.

6. Rainer Maria Rilke, *Letters to a Young Poet*, trans. M. D. Herter Norton (repr., W. W. Norton, 2004), 27.

Chapter 3 This Is for the Truth-Teller

1. Kaytee Gillis, "8 Common Dysfunctional Family Roles: Through Self-Awareness, We Can Work to Change Patterns We Took into Adulthood," *Psychology Today*, March 23, 2023, https://www.psychologytoday.com/us/blog/invisible-bruises/202303/8-common-dysfunctional-family-roles.

2. Herbert Goldenberg and Irene Goldenberg, *Family Therapy: An Overview*, 7th ed. (Thomson Higher Education, 2008), 244.

3. Peter A. Levine and Maggie Kline, *Trauma Through a Child's Eyes: Awakening the Ordinary Miracle of Healing* (North Atlantic Books, 2007), 30.

4. Anne Lamott, *Plan B: Further Thoughts on Faith* (Riverhead Books, 2006), 174.

5. Holly Whitaker, *Quit Like a Woman: The Radical Choice to Not Drink in a Culture Obsessed with Alcohol* (Dial Press, 2019), 148.

Chapter 5 Find Your Edges

1. Online Etymology Dictionary, "dissociate," accessed September 12, 2024, https://www.etymonline.com/word/dissociate.

2. "What Are Dissociative Disorders?" American Psychiatric Association, accessed August 1, 2024, https://www.psychiatry.org/patients-families/dissociative-disorders/what-are-dissociative-disorders.

3. James W. Pennebaker and Joshua M. Smyth, *Opening Up by Writing It Down: How Expressive Writing Improves Health and Eases Emotional Pain* (Guilford Press, 2016), 9.

4. Pete Walker, "The 4Fs: A Trauma Typology in Complex PTSD," Pete Walker, M.A., MFT, accessed August 1, 2024, https://www.pete-walker.com/fourFs_TraumaTypologyComplexPTSD.htm.

5. Jackee Holder, "Non-Dominant Hand Writing Therapy," *Psychologies*, March 17, 2022, https://www.psychologies.co.uk/non-dominant-hand-writing-therapy.

Chapter 6 Creative Consensuality

1. Daniel J. Siegel, *The Developing Mind: How Relationships and the Brain Interact to Shape Who We Are*, 3rd ed. (Guilford Press, 2020).

2. Merriam-Webster, "deadline," accessed July 29, 2024, https://www.merriam-webster.com/dictionary/deadline.

3. Merriam-Webster, "lifeline," accessed July 30, 2024, https://www.merriam-webster.com/dictionary/lifeline.

4. Merriam-Webster, "the bends," accessed August 5, 2024, https://www.merriam-webster.com/dictionary/the%20bends.

Chapter 7 Eyes on the Horizon

1. Stephanie Manes, "Making Sure Emotional Flooding Doesn't Capsize Your Relationship," The Gottman Institute, accessed August 1, 2024, https://www.gottman.com/blog/making-sure-emotional-flooding-doesnt-capsize-your-relationship/.

Chapter 8 Can I Get a Word Witness?

1. Online Etymology Dictionary, "witness," accessed September 12, 2024, https://www.etymonline.com/word/witness.

2. See Luke 22:44.

3. H. R. Jerajani, Bhagyashri Jaju, M. M. Phiske, and Nitin Lade, "Hematohidrosis: A Rare Clinical Phenomenon," *Indian Journal of Dermatology* 54, no. 3 (Jul–Sep 2009): 290–92, https://www.ncbi.nlm.nih.gov/pmc/articles/PMC2810702/.

4. Matthew 26:38 CEV.

5. John 20:27 NIV.

Chapter 9 Welcome Home, Prodigal Writer

1. Madeleine L'Engle, *A Circle of Quiet* (HarperSanFrancisco, 1984), 199–200.
2. See Luke 15:11–32.

Chapter 10 Inner Child Altars

1. Elinor Greenberg, "How to Use Gestalt Therapy to Interpret Dreams," *Psychology Today*, April 1, 2023, https://www.psychologytoday.com/us/blog /understanding-narcissism/202304/how-to-use-gestalt-therapy-to-inter pret-dreams.
2. Encyclopedia.com, "altar," accessed September 12, 2024, https://www .encyclopedia.com/philosophy-and-religion/other-religious-beliefs-and -general-terms/religion-general/altar.
3. John O'Donohue, *To Bless the Space Between Us: A Book of Blessings* (Doubleday, 2008), 198, 199.

Chapter 11 Passing Through Grief Portals

1. Shelly Rambo, *Spirit and Trauma: A Theology of Remaining* (Westminster John Knox, 2010), 7.
2. Suzanne Phillips, "'The Space Between 'What Was' and 'What's Next': The Liminal Space," PsychCentral, March 22, 2017, https://psychcentral .com/blog/healing-together/2017/03/the-space-between-what-was-and -whats-next-the-liminal-space#1.
3. Whole Health Library, "Grief Reactions, Duration, and Tasks of Mourning," U.S. Department of Veterans Affairs, accessed August 8, 2024, https://www.va.gov/WHOLEHEALTHLIBRARY/tools/grief-reactions-du ration-and-tasks-of-mourning.asp. See also J. William Worden, *Grief Counseling and Grief Therapy: A Handbook for the Mental Health Practitioner*, 4th ed. (Springer, 2008).
4. Roxane Gay, *Writing into the Wound: Understanding Trauma, Truth, and Language* (Scribd Originals, 2021), 37.
5. "What Is a Prayer Labyrinth?" Got Questions, accessed August 8, 2024, https://www.gotquestions.org/prayer-labyrinth.html.
6. Parker J. Palmer, *Let Your Life Speak: Listening for the Voice of Vocation*, 25th anniv. ed. (Jossey-Bass, 2024), 27.

Chapter 12 Your Body Is Brilliant

1. Stephen Winick, "Ring Around the Rosie: Metafolklore, Rhyme and Reason," *Folklife Today* (blog), July 24, 2014, https://blogs.loc.gov/folklife /2014/07/ring-around-the-rosie-metafolklore-rhyme-and-reason/.

2. Alice Miller, *The Body Never Lies: The Lingering Effects of Hurtful Parenting*, trans. Andrew Jenkins (W. W. Norton, 2005), 19.

3. Annie G. Rogers, *The Unsayable: The Hidden Language of Trauma* (Ballantine Books, 2007), xiv.

Chapter 13 Becoming the Good Samaritan of Your Stories

1. Jalal al-Din Rumi, "The Guest House," in *The Essential Rumi*, rev. ed., trans. Coleman Barks with John Moyne, A. J. Arberry, and Reynold Nicholson (HarperCollins, 2004), 109.

2. Luke 10:30–34 VOICE.

Chapter 14 Writing Through Attachment Styles

1. Steven Pressfield, *The War of Art: Break Through the Blocks and Win Your Inner Creative Battles* (Black Irish Entertainment, 2012), 40.

2. Inge Bretherton, "The Origins of Attachment Theory: John Bowlby and Mary Ainsworth," *Developmental Psychology* 28, no. 5 (1992): 759–75, https://doi.org/10.1037/0012-1649.28.5.759.

3. Kendra Cherry, "What Is Attachment Theory?: The Importance of Early Emotional Bonds," Verywell Mind, accessed August 8, 2024, https://www.verywellmind.com/what-is-attachment-theory-2795337.

4. D. W. Winnicott, *Playing and Reality*, Routledge Classics ed. (Routledge, 2005), 13.

5. Annie Dillard, *The Writing Life* (HarperCollins, 1989), 52.

Chapter 15 Rebuilding After the Rupture

1. John Bowlby, "Attachment Theory and Its Therapeutic Implications," *Adolescent Psychiatry* 6 (1978): 5–33.

Chapter 16 We Can't Outrun Our Stories

1. Raymond Bernard Blakney, ed., *Meister Eckhart: A Modern Translation* (Harper & Row, 1941), 9.

Closing Thoughts

1. Judith Lewis Herman, *Trauma and Recovery: The Aftermath of Violence—From Domestic Abuse to Political Terror* (Basic Books, 1992), 133.

MEGAN FEBUARY is an author, trauma-informed writing coach, editor, and leading expert in creative recovery. Her teachings on the body as a storyteller have supported hundreds at story workshops and writing retreats. As the founder of the literary magazine *For Women Who Roar* and her specialized writing programs, Megan has guided thousands of women through the process of writing, healing their stories, and releasing them into the world. At a young age, she came to writing and creativity to heal her own trauma and has dedicated her life to helping others do the same. Over the years, she has been called a master guide for all things writing and creativity and has been praised even by the queen of creativity herself, Julia Cameron, author of *The Artist's Way*, who called her work "powerful and far-seeing." Megan currently resides in the Pacific Northwest and is writing her next book.